The Athletic Trainer's Guide to Differential Diagnosis

A Visual Learning Approach

The Athletic Trainer's Guide to Differential Diagnosis

A Visual Learning Approach

Andrew P. Winterstein, PhD, ATC
Clinical Professor
Athletic Training Program Director
University of Wisconsin—Madison

Sharon V. Clark, MS, ATC
Associate Faculty
Athletic Training Program Clinical Coordinator
University of Wisconsin—Madison

Routledge
Taylor & Francis Group
NEW YORK AND LONDON

First published in hardback 2024

First published in 2015 by SLACK Incorporated

Published 2024 by Routledge
605 Third Avenue, New York, NY 10058

and by Routledge
4 Park Square, Milton Park, Abingdon, Oxon OX14 4RN

Routledge is an imprint of the Taylor & Francis Group, an informa business

Andrew P. Winterstein and Sharon V. Clark have no financial or proprietary interest in the materials presented herein.

Publisher's Note
The publisher has gone to great lengths to ensure the quality of this reprint but points out that some imperfections in the original copies may be apparent.

Library of Congress Cataloging-in-Publication Data

Winterstein, Andrew P., 1962- author.
The athletic trainer's guide to differential diagnosis : a visual learning approach / Andrew P. Winterstein, Sharon V. Clark.
p. ; cm.
Includes bibliographical references and index.

I. Clark, Sharon V., 1965- author. II. Title.
[DNLM: 1. Athletic Injuries--diagnosis--Case Reports. 2. Diagnosis, Differential--Case Reports. 3. Diagnostic Techniques and Procedures--Case Reports. QT 261]
RD97
617.1'027--dc23

2014018257

ISBN: 978-1-03-296440-9 (hbk)
ISBN: 978-1-61711-053-5 (pbk)
ISBN: 978-1-003-52265-2 (ebk)

DOI: 10.4324/9781003522652

Dedication

This book is dedicated to all of the students, clinical preceptors, physicians, and faculty who help make the Athletic Training Program at UW-Madison something special.

This book is also dedicated to my mom, Pat Winterstein (for hanging tough), to my sister Michele (for all you do), and to all the Winterstein gang (just because).

And always, Barb.

Andrew P. Winterstein, PhD, ATC

I would like to dedicate this book to all the students who have challenged me to become a better educator, and to Andy for making this project happen and his innovative teaching strategies that have inspired me to think outside the box. I especially want to thank my husband, Brent, daughter, Carly, and son, Luke, for their love, support, and encouragement throughout the writing process. You are the reason I strive to be the best I can be every day.

Sharon V. Clark, MS, ATC

Contents

Acknowledgments

The process of taking on a large project is very much like a road trip; you may start out with a map, but ultimately you just have to find your way. Book projects are filled with equal parts excitement and trepidation, with plenty of uncertainty tossed in along the way; yet, if you stick with them, you get the satisfaction of seeing the final product. However, anyone who has ever taken such a trip knows that you need plenty of help along the way. It is in that spirit that we need to say thank you to some people who made the journey much more pleasant and kept us on the right road.

Ms. Lindsay Donath is a wonderful young athletic trainer and physical therapist with a fabulous career ahead of her. She was instrumental in moving many parts of this project forward and her efforts were invaluable. We appreciate her work ethic and dependability; her future patients will be in great hands.

We also wish to thank Ms. Linda Endlich from the University of Wisconsin MERIT library for her assistance in designing the figures and templates for this project. Her graphic design skills are exceptional and her patience with a novice InDesign user is greatly appreciated.

We would like to thank the staff at SLACK Incorporated (past and present) who had a hand in this project: Jennifer Briggs, Brien Cummings, Michelle Gatt, April Billick, John Bond, Jordyn Bennett, and anyone who assisted with the editing, layout, and production. We appreciate your efforts on our behalf.

A big thanks to the staff at Barriques on Monroe Street in Madison for the gallons of vanilla black tea, plenty of cowboy cookies, and allowing us to set up shop to write on a regular basis.

Lastly, we would like to thank our spouses and families for their encouragement and patience during this journey; your support and love mean the most.

Acknowledgments

About the Authors

Andrew P. Winterstein, PhD, ATC is a clinical professor in the Department of Kinesiology at the University of Wisconsin–Madison in Madison, Wisconsin, where he serves as the program director of their CAATE-accredited athletic training professional preparation program. He also maintains an affiliate appointment in the Department of Orthopedics and Rehabilitation in the School of Medicine and Public Health. Dr. Winterstein has been at the University of Wisconsin since 1986. He provided clinical care as part of the athletic training staff in the Division of Intercollegiate Athletics for 14 years before moving over to direct the AT education program. He is an alumnus of the University of Arizona in Tucson, Arizona, University of Oregon in Eugene, Oregon, and the University of Wisconsin–Madison.

Dr. Winterstein's academic interests include studying emerging technologies and their use in teaching and learning; medical humanities and their application to athletic training education; organizational dynamics and behaviors; patient outcomes following injury; and the Scholarship of Teaching and Learning (SoTL). His papers and abstracts have appeared in the *Journal of Athletic Training, Athletic Therapy Today, Sports Health,* and *Athletic Training and Sports Health Care.* He has been privileged to make numerous professional presentations at the state, regional, and national level.

A certified member of the National Athletic Trainers' Association since 1985 and a certified member of the Wisconsin Athletic Trainers' Association, Dr. Winterstein is active in many aspects of athletic training. He serves as a reviewer for the *Journal of Athletic Training* and the *Athletic Training Education Journal,* is a reviewer and member of the editorial board for *Athletic Training and Sports Health Care,* and has served on several state, regional, and national committees. Dr. Winterstein has received numerous awards, including the 2008 Great Lakes Athletic Training Association Outstanding Educator Award, the 2007 Wisconsin Athletic Trainers Association Outstanding Educator Award, and the 2006 University of Wisconsin–Madison School of Education Distinguished Service Award. He and his colleagues were three-time winners of the NATA Educational Multimedia Committee award for educational innovations and have been awarded the MERLOT Classics Award for exemplary on-line learning objects. He is the author of two textbooks, *The Athletic Training Student Primer* (now in its 2nd edition) and *Administrative Topics in Athletic Training: Concepts to Practice* (coauthored with Gary L. Harrelson, EdD, ATC and Greg Gardner, EdD, ATC, LAT), both published by SLACK Incorporated.

In his spare time, Andy enjoys fly fishing, stand-up paddle boarding, reading, and writing. He resides in Madison, Wisconsin with his wife, Barb.

Sharon V. Clark, MS, ATC is an assistant faculty associate in the Department of Kinesiology at the University of Wisconsin–Madison in Madison, Wisconsin, where she currently serves as Clinical Coordinator and instructor in their CAATE-accredited professional preparation program in athletic training. She also maintains a position as a senior athletic trainer for the Sports Rehabilitation Physical Therapy and Athletic Training Department of UWHealth. She continues to participate in outreach athletic training event coverage for UWHealth. Ms. Clark has been with the University of Wisconsin–Madison since 2009, and has been a care provider for UWHealth for over 18 years. Prior to working in the rehabilitation clinical setting, she provided athletic training services as a physician extender and at an area high school. Ms. Clark is an alumnus of the University of Wisconsin-Madison.

In her spare time, Ms. Clark enjoys running, kayaking, and following her children in their respective activities. She resides in Madison, Wisconsin with her husband, Brent, and two children, Carly and Luke.

Foreword

The Athletic Trainer's Guide to Differential Diagnosis: A Visual Learning Approach, authored by Andrew P. Winterstein and Sharon V. Clark, is an excellent addition to the athletic trainer's library. The active learning approach is perhaps nontraditional, in that a visual mapping approach to the differential diagnosis of a wide variety of clinical problems provides a rather novel and refreshing way to aid the athletic trainer in day-to-day clinical practice. Twelve chapters, each covering a different body part, are delivered in a systematic fashion that includes a general introduction, followed by a case study, and differential diagnosis map that includes the traditional history, injury mechanism, key findings, and diagnostic evidence.

Students and practicing athletic trainers alike will find this study guide quite helpful. The detailed and meticulous approach to the time-honored differential diagnosis in a unique fashion is stimulating. The addition of this cutting-edge method is long overdue, and will put athletic trainers in a unique perspective amongst other healthcare providers. The presentation is logical, the illustrations are appropriately detailed, and the differential diagnosis is presented, not in a "how to," but rather a "what if" approach to common clinical problems confronting the athletic trainer.

In this reference guide, the authors have moved the sports medicine field forward. The subject matter is referenced in a scholarly, up-to-date manner that provides an added benefit to those fortunate enough to have access to this material. The logical flow of this text, with a particular focus on the differential diagnosis, is a testament to the commitment of the authors to improve the care of athletes by ensuring best practice in a comprehensive and novel way. It is now up to the reader to act on the approach using the information provided!

Thomas Best, MD, PhD
Ohio State University
Columbus, Ohio

1

How to Use This Guide/The Learning Diagram Approach

Determining the nature and severity of a diagnosis seems straightforward enough. Collect the pertinent history, perform the proper components of the physical exam, think critically about the information in front of you, and commit to a diagnosis. However, the ability to make that commitment to a diagnosis is one of the most difficult steps for clinicians in training; there are so many possibilities. Students need to consider all the available injuries and conditions, not to mention the various diagnostic elements that must be remembered and applied correctly. A clear and logical approach is needed to avoid getting mired down in the process. Most of us can learn all the proper skills that go into the evaluation and, with practice, the right questions to ask in the history and the proper special tests and physical exam components become second nature. However, putting the pieces together and knowing what possibilities lay at the end of the evaluation process is what separates the mere technician from a true, independent clinician. *The Athletic Trainer's Guide to Differential Diagnosis: A Visual Learning Approach* provides a way of thinking that helps the reader sort through the possibilities and think about the clinical evaluation within a structured framework using a visual mapping approach.

Differential diagnosis is defined as *the determination of which of two or more conditions with similar signs and symptoms is the one from which the patient is suffering, by a systematic comparison and contrasting of the clinical findings.*[1] The key phrase in this definition is "a systematic comparison and contrasting of the clinical findings." The visual mapping approach outlined

Winterstein AP, Clark SV. *The Athletic Trainer's Guide to Differential Diagnosis (pp 1-4).*

in this guide provides a visual systematic framework for identifying possible diagnoses. Each chapter provides a general introduction, followed by a case study or "paper patient." An artistic interpretation of the anatomy for each region is presented to allow for general orientation. The differential diagnosis map for each body part is presented and organized by primary location of symptoms (eg, anterior, posterior, lateral, and medial). The clinical findings for each condition outlined on the map are provided, including history, mechanism of injury, testing, key findings, and diagnostic evidence. Diagnostic evidence is presented in the form by references to specific literature, diagnostic clinical correlations, and presentation of sensitivity and specificity data for specific tests. Specificity refers to the ability of a clinical test to correctly identify patients with a condition. Sensitivity refers to the ability of a clinical test to correctly identify those patients without a condition.[2] This information allows the reader to review the differential diagnosis map for each body part and compare and contrast the various findings.

The practice of mapping the various possibilities is a useful learning skill for students. Seeing the visual map allows the learner to consider the possible diagnoses by location and approach the evaluation in a more focused and organized fashion. This approach will allow for more efficient clinical evaluations, will advance clinical reasoning skills, and avoid a shotgun approach. Practicing clinicians can employ this method to help organize their thoughts and to fully consider possible diagnoses when faced with difficult cases. The visual mapping method of evaluation also allows the reader the opportunity to apply evidence-based principles to the clinical evaluation process. Users of this manual will develop critical thinking skills and will have ample opportunity to integrate information from previous courses. *The Athletic Trainer's Guide to Differential Diagnosis* is not designed as a "how-to" evaluation text. This guide is designed to create a framework that allows the reader to think differently about differential diagnoses, access existing knowledge in anatomy and clinical evaluation, and assess information for the purpose of making higher-order clinical decisions.

Clinical Learning: Memorizing Is Not Enough!

Instructors often like to challenge students with the questions:

- How do you know what you know?
- Where did that knowledge come from?

Consider a relatively simple injury evaluation. Let's say you have a patient who is a recreational runner and you have diagnosed him or her with pes anserine bursitis. You are confident in your findings, but we need to proceed with care:

- How do we know that is what the patient has?
- Can you defend the diagnosis?
- What information brought you to that conclusion?
- What else could it be?
- How did you rule those possibilities out?

Somewhere along the way, you acquired some knowledge about, in this case, pes anserine bursitis. You must have learned the anatomy, the three tendons that make up the pes group, and maybe you learned the word origin of *pes* (Latin for foot or foot-like part) that helps describe the tendons. Somewhere you learned what types of patients might have pes anserine bursitis. At some point, you learned what factors might predispose a patient to this condition. It is also important to know what other conditions you should consider when diagnosing this problem and what the typical findings are for this condition so you can perform a complete evaluation. The point is this: it is doubtful you learned all of this at once.

When we learn, we must access knowledge that we already have along with new information that we acquire. This, in turn, helps us create a new foundation of knowledge. It is from this evolving foundation of knowledge that we approach new problems. It really is quite simple. We tend to build knowledge and knowledge tends to change. Yes, the knowledge tends to change. Injury evaluation and diagnosis changes because we are constantly learning new ways to apply special tests, and discovering new evidence about which tests are most effective. As diagnostic tools improve, we can better correlate our clinical findings with advanced imaging and surgical correlates. It never stops. As learners (hopefully the lifelong kind), we need to be open to the idea of always adding to this foundation of knowledge.

Thinking about evaluation and diagnosis makes me think about detective stories; each injury evaluation is like a detective's case that needs to be solved. There are things we can see, information we need from the patient, tests we can perform, and then we have to put all the pieces together to come to a defensible conclusion. It is this "putting the pieces together" that can only occur with clinical practice and a constantly evolving foundation of knowledge. Students can only learn the subtleties and nuances of injury evaluation through practice that takes place on a foundation of knowledge, and that foundation cannot be static. Processing and synthesizing information to come to a logical conclusion represents higher-order thinking. Because this thinking requires the hands-on application of skills with live patients, it cannot only be learned in a book—it must be practiced. The goals of this guide are to provide a framework for that practice, and to motivate the student to take the information from the page into clinical practice.

How to Use This Guide

We hope that this book can serve as a spark for active learning. Our goal is to provide the reader with an incentive to use the tools in this guide to help reinforce current knowledge and add to that evolving foundation of knowledge. In the interest of active learning, we encourage readers to:

- Practice by using the case studies in the guide
- Utilize the templates in Appendix A to draw their own differential diagnosis maps
- Make use of the clinical findings templates in Appendix B to work through individual injuries and conditions
- Take the mapping skills and framework for thinking about differential diagnosis into their own clinical learning and clinical practice

In short, we want our readers to be active learners and keep constructing their own knowledge. We hope this guide proves helpful as readers develop and refine their clinical skills.

References

1. Merriam-Webster.com. 2014. http://www.merriam-webster.com/medlineplus (Accessed June 2, 2014).
2. Lalkhen AG, McCluskey A. Clinical tests: sensitivity and specificity. *Contin Educ Anaesth Crit Care Pain.* 2008;8(6):221-223.

2

The Foot

As a species that walks upright and relies on bipedal motion, the foot has taken on added importance in our evolution. The foot provides a stable base at the distal end of our lower extremity; aids in attenuating forces when we walk, run, and land; and acts as a rigid lever during the push off portion of our gait cycle.[1] Injuries to the foot are fairly common in sports and recreational activity. In a study of lower extremity injury patterns in high school athletes in 2005, Fernandez et al[2] found that the foot represented 7.1% of all injuries and 18% of all fractures. A 1-year query of foot injuries related to sport and recreation among teens revealed that over 25,000 teens report to emergency rooms with foot injuries annually, and these represent about 4% of the total sports injuries that present to emergency rooms annually.[3] Ascertaining injury rates for the foot can be difficult because many studies report foot injuries in combination with data on ankle injuries.[4]

The foot is made up of 26 bones (7 tarsal bones, 5 metatarsal bones, and 14 bones that make up the phalanges). Anatomically, the foot can be divided into 3 regions: rearfoot (posterior segment), midfoot (middle segment), and forefoot (anterior segment). Each of these segments has a variety of articulations. Coupled with the array of bony articulations is a complex network of superficial tendons, bursa, retinaculum, nerve, and facial tissue that is susceptible to a variety of mechanical forces and subsequent injury. The foot is susceptible to acute trauma through compression ("stepped on") injuries and to injury mechanisms that cause sprain injuries. A host of injury mechanisms common to the ankle (eg, inversion, eversion, and

Winterstein AP, Clark SV. *The Athletic Trainer's Guide to Differential Diagnosis (pp 5-33).*

rotation) can also cause injury to the foot. Clinicians must differentiate foot and ankle injuries with care.

The diagnostic maps for the foot have been divided into 4 regions: dorsal (top of the foot), plantar (bottom of the foot), medial, and lateral. This allows for thoughtful mapping of the injuries to the foot to better delineate possible diagnoses for the clinician.

Paper Patient: Foot Pain in a Runner

History

Sarah is a 30-year-old runner who noticed pain in her left foot 10 weeks ago. She took 2 weeks off from running and treated her foot with ice and ibuprofen. She felt better and started running again. After running for 2 weeks, she still had pain, so she took 4 weeks off and wore a night splint to bed. She had been training for a half marathon, but now she is worried she has missed too much training time. Sarah describes a pain (4/10) in her foot that runs from the heel through the mid arch to her forefoot. She also notices pain (2/10) in the upper part of her heel near the Achilles insertion. She has a history of foot/ankle pain with training for a half marathon in the past, but she did not seek care. She does have some first step pain upon waking, but not every day.

Physical Exam

Observation of Sarah's feet in both standing and walking gait reveal mild pes planus and rear foot valgus. She is tender to palpation over the plantar fascia at medial calcaneal tubercle and over a broad area of tissue at the mid portion of the longitudinal arch. There is no bony tenderness noted on exam. Active range of motion (AROM) of the ankle is within normal limits (WNL) and pain free. Passive range of motion (PROM) is WNL and pain free with normal end feel; tightness of the posterior leg musculature is noted. She has pain with resisted flexion and extension of her toes. She also has pain with palpation along the medial arch to the great toe. Her neurovascular exam is normal.

Clinical Decisions

- What is your differential diagnosis?
- What keys do you see with this case to help with your differentials?

Start with a review of the anatomy map and consider the possible injuries and conditions that are common to the foot. Use the differential diagnosis maps of the foot to guide your thought process and organize the possibilities. We will revisit this case at the end of the chapter.

Anatomy Map: Foot

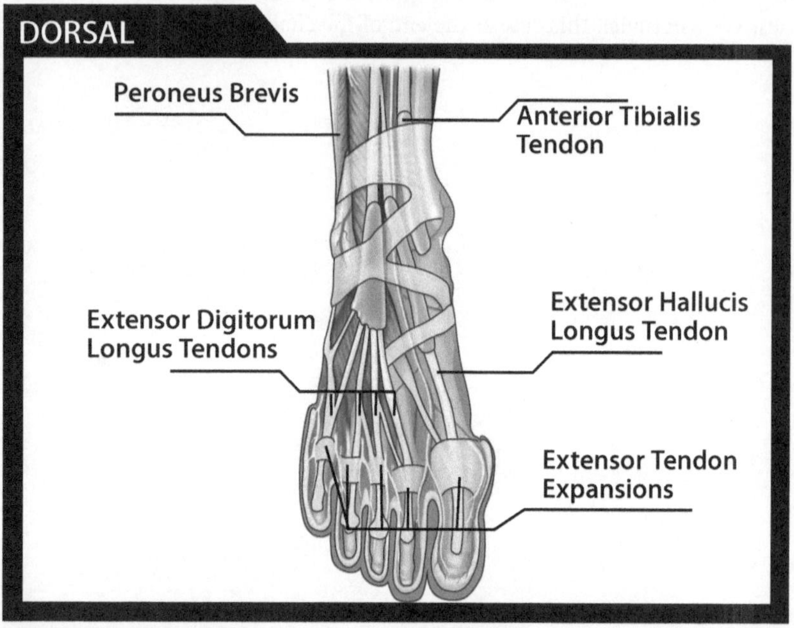

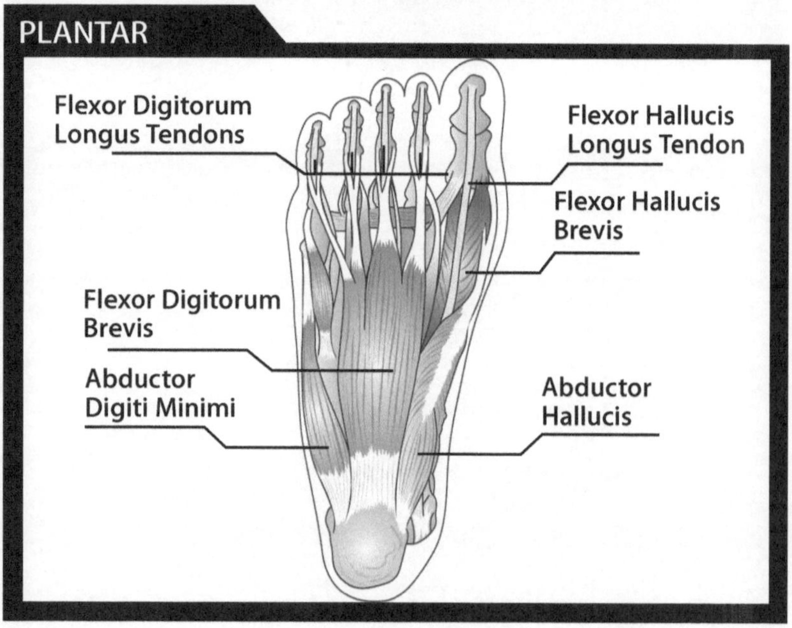

Anatomy Map: Foot

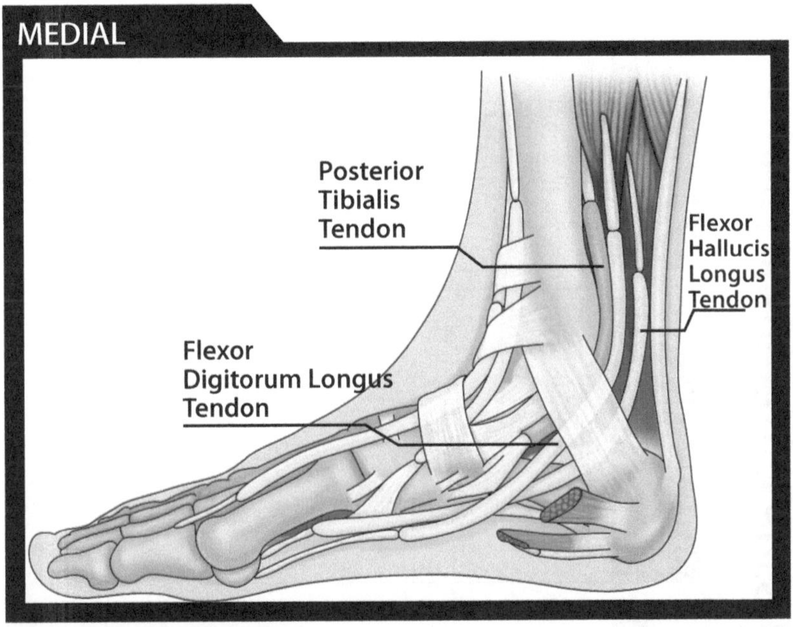

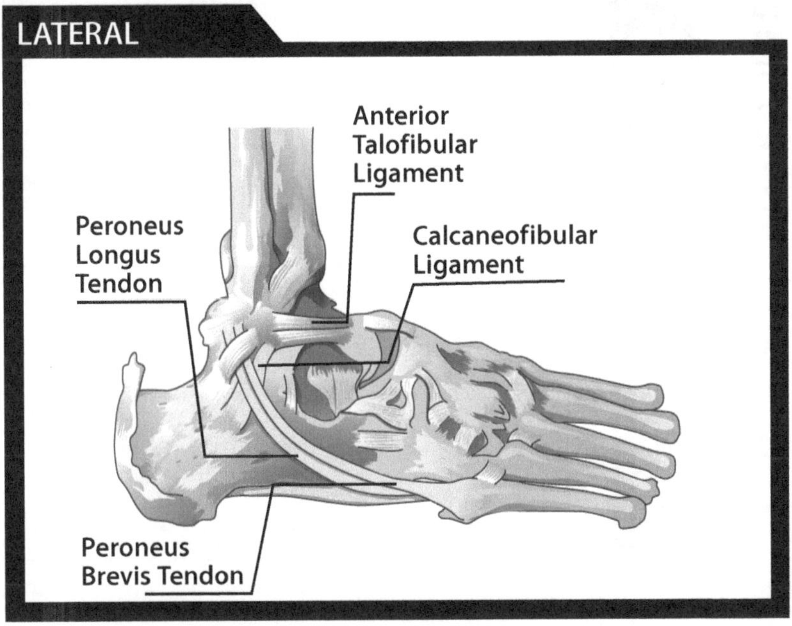

Foot Map: Region/Soft Tissue Differential Diagnosis

DORSAL

- Extensor Digitorum Tendinopathy
- Extensor Hallicus Tendinopathy
- Hallux Rigidus
- Interphalangeal (IP) Sprain
- Lisfranc Sprain
- Metatarsalgia
- Midfoot Sprain
- Tibialis Anterior Tendinopathy

PLANTAR

- Flexor Digitorum Tendinopathy
- Flexor Hallicus Tendinopathy
- Morton's Neuroma
- Plantar Fasciitis
- Sesamoiditis

MEDIAL

- First Metatarso-phalangeal (MTP) Sprain (Turf Toe)
- Hallux Valgus Deformity/Bunion/ Exostosis
- Tarsal Tunnel Syndrome
- Posterior Tibialis Tendinopathy

LATERAL

- Bunionette or Tailor's Bunion
- Cuboid Subluxation Syndrome
- Peroneal Tendinopathy

Foot Pain

Injuries to Bone/Joint Surfaces

COMMON FRACTURES

- Avulsion fracture of the fifth metatarsal (peroneus brevis)
- Base of the fifth metatatarsal (Jones)
- Calcaneal fracture
- Cuboid fracture
- Metatarsal fracture
- Metatarsal stress fracture
- Navicular stress fracture
- Phalangeal fracture

Note: Stress fractures can result from mechanical loading factors and/or metabolic issues leading to insufficiency in bone health. Careful consideration must be given to patient history, activity level, and bone health. Stress fractures to the foot are common and must be referred for appropriate follow up.

Clinical Assessment of Foot Injuries

Dorsal Foot Pain

Extensor Digitorum Tendinopathy

HISTORY	MECHANISM OF INJURY	EVALUATION ESSENTIALS
• Patient reports pain on top of the foot • Patient may see swelling on top of foot • Patient may describe changes in training volume or intensity	• Poor footwear • Excessive tightness of the calf complex	• Palpation of the extensor digitorum • Range of motion (ROM) testing • Manual muscle testing (MMT) of the extensor digitorum

KEY FINDINGS	DIAGNOSTIC EVIDENCE
• Pain reproduced with MMT • Pain is specific to the second to fifth digits	• Magnetic resonance imaging (MRI) can be useful to identify edema and inflammatory changes • Ultrasound can detect thickening of the tendon and assess the gliding ability of the tendon through specific ROM[5]

Dorsal Foot Pain

Extensor Hallucis Tendinopathy

HISTORY	MECHANISM OF INJURY	EVALUATION ESSENTIALS
• Patient reports pain on top of the foot • Patient may see swelling on top of foot • Patient may describe changes in training volume or intensity	• Poor footwear • Excessive tightness of the calf complex	• Palpation of the extensor hallucis • ROM testing • MMT of the extensor hallucis

KEY FINDINGS	DIAGNOSTIC EVIDENCE
• Pain reproduced with MMT • Pain is specific to the great toe	• MRI can be useful to identify edema and inflammatory changes • Ultrasound can detect thickening of the tendon and assess the gliding ability of the tendon through specific ROM[5]

Dorsal Foot Pain

Hallux Rigidus

HISTORY	MECHANISM OF INJURY	EVALUATION ESSENTIALS
• Patient reports pain at the first MTP joint • Patient describes stiffness or the inability to flex and extend at the first MTP • Patient describes difficulty with push off	• Prior trauma to first MTP • Family history	• Palpation of the first MTP • ROM testing • Radiograph

KEY FINDINGS	DIAGNOSTIC EVIDENCE
• True etiology is unknown • More common in females than males aged 30 to 60 • May have swelling of joint with bone spur formation	• A four-stage radiographic classification system has been developed to aid in conservative and surgical management[6]

Dorsal Foot Pain

Interphalangeal Sprain

HISTORY	MECHANISM OF INJURY	EVALUATION ESSENTIALS
• Patient reports pain at the IP joint • Patient describes stiffness at the IP joint	• Sudden hyperextension injury • Sudden hyperflexion injury	• Palpation of the IP joint • ROM testing • Radiograph

KEY FINDINGS	DIAGNOSTIC EVIDENCE
• Most commonly an acute injury • Occasionally from a repetitive stress • May have swelling of the joint	• No diagnostic evidence available

Dorsal Foot Pain

Lisfranc Sprain

HISTORY	MECHANISM OF INJURY	EVALUATION ESSENTIALS
• Patient reports pain in the midfoot • Patient describes pain that increases with standing or walking	• Simple twist and fall with a plantarflexed foot • Trauma from fall • Forced trauma on plantarflexed foot (eg, opponent lands on foot)	• Palpation of the midfoot • ROM testing • Stabilize calcaneus and rotate the midfoot • Flexion and extension of the digits • Raise on tip toes • Radiograph/MRI/computed tomography (CT)

KEY FINDINGS	DIAGNOSTIC EVIDENCE
• Need to rule out Lisfranc fracture from ligament sprain • Occasionally from a repetitive stress • May see swelling and ecchymosis of both dorsal and plantar aspect of foot	• Radiographs are often inconclusive, causing the MRI to become the gold standard for evaluating surrounding ligamentous and bony structures[7]

Dorsal Foot Pain

Metatarsalgia

HISTORY	MECHANISM OF INJURY	EVALUATION ESSENTIALS
• Patient reports pain at the metatarsals either just the first digit or digits 2 to 4 • Patient describes sharp, aching, or burning pain • Patient has no pain with rest and increased pain with weight bearing activities	• Increased training • Poorly fitting footwear	• Palpation of the metatarsals at the MTP joints • ROM testing • Metatarsal squeeze testing

KEY FINDINGS	DIAGNOSTIC EVIDENCE
• May develop suddenly with increased training; most develop over time • Foot type (hallux valgus, pes cavus and hammer toes) and body weight also play a factor	• Radiographs or MRI may be warranted to rule out stress fractures[8]

Dorsal Foot Pain

Midfoot Sprain

HISTORY	MECHANISM OF INJURY	EVALUATION ESSENTIALS
• Patient reports pain in the midfoot • Patient describes pain that increases with standing or walking	• Isolated twisting • Trauma from fall • Collision	• Palpation of the midfoot • ROM testing • Stabilize calcaneus and rotate the midfoot • Radiograph/MRI/CT

KEY FINDINGS	DIAGNOSTIC EVIDENCE
• Palpation and testing will be specific for the specific area of sprain • May see swelling and ecchymosis	• Radiographs are often inconclusive, causing the MRI to become the gold standard for evaluating surrounding ligamentous and bony structures[7]

Dorsal Foot Pain

Tibialis Anterior Tendinopathy

HISTORY	MECHANISM OF INJURY	EVALUATION ESSENTIALS
• Patient reports pain at the insertion of the tibialis anterior • Patient describes pain in the morning • Patient has no pain with rest and increased pain with weight bearing activities	• Increased training • Footwear that is too tight over the tibialis anterior	• Palpation of the insertion of the tibialis anterior • ROM testing • MMT for the tibialis anterior

KEY FINDINGS	DIAGNOSTIC EVIDENCE
• May develop suddenly with increased training; most develop over time	• MRI can be useful to identify edema and inflammatory changes • Ultrasound can detect thickening of the tendon and assess the gliding ability of the tendon through specific ROM[5]

Plantar Foot Pain

Flexor Digitorum Tendinopathy

HISTORY	MECHANISM OF INJURY	EVALUATION ESSENTIALS
• Patient reports pain on the bottom of the foot • Patient may describe swelling on bottom of foot	• Repetitive plantarflexion • Traumatic	• Palpation of the flexor digitorum • ROM testing • MMT of the flexor digitorum

KEY FINDINGS	DIAGNOSTIC EVIDENCE
• Pain reproduced with MMT • Pain is specific to the second to the fifth digits	• MRI can be useful to identify edema and inflammatory changes • Ultrasound can detect thickening of the tendon and assess the gliding ability of the tendon through specific ROM[5]

Plantar Foot Pain

Flexor Hallucis Tendinopathy

HISTORY	MECHANISM OF INJURY	EVALUATION ESSENTIALS
• Patient reports pain on the bottom of the foot • Patient may see swelling on the bottom of foot	• Traumatic • Repetitive plantarflexion	• Palpation of the flexor hallucis • ROM testing • MMT of the flexor hallucis

KEY FINDINGS	DIAGNOSTIC EVIDENCE
• Pain reproduced with MMT • Pain is specific to the great toe • The flexor hallucis longus helps maintain the arch	• MRI can be useful to identify edema and inflammatory changes • Ultrasound can detect thickening of the tendon and assess the gliding ability of the tendon through specific ROM[5]

Plantar Foot Pain

Morton's Neuroma

HISTORY	MECHANISM OF INJURY	EVALUATION ESSENTIALS
• Patient reports pain on the bottom of the foot • Patient describes a feeling of walking on a pebble in the ball of the foot • Patient may experience numbness and tingling in the toes	• Repetitive irritation or pressure to nerve • Traumatic injury to nerve	• Palpation of the metatarsal area specifically between the third and fourth metatarsals • ROM testing • Squeeze test of the metatarsal heads reproducing the symptoms

KEY FINDINGS	DIAGNOSTIC EVIDENCE
• Wearing high heels and foot deformities are risk factors • Avoid shoes with narrow toe box; adjusting lacing pattern of athletic shoes may cause relief • Sometimes will see this between the second and third metatarsals	• MRI (sensitivity 88%) and ultrasonography (sensitivity 96%) can be used to confirm presence of neuroma[9]

Plantar Foot Pain

Plantar Fasciitis

HISTORY	MECHANISM OF INJURY	EVALUATION ESSENTIALS
• Patient reports having heel pain • Patient describes difficulty with walking • Patient complains of pain that is greatest with first steps in the morning or after prolonged sitting	• Rapid increase in activity combined with poor foot wear • Repetitive irritation in the form of tension of the plantar aponeurosis	• Palpation of the medial calcaneal tubercle • ROM testing

KEY FINDINGS	DIAGNOSTIC EVIDENCE
• Pes cavus hypomobile foot • Pes planus hypermobile foot • Tightness of the gastrocnemius and soleus unit common • Patient may have a heel spur visible on radiograph • Palpable crepitus along the plantar aspect of the foot in many patients	• Ankle dorsiflexion for gastrocnemius and soleus tightness (sensitivity 100%, specificity 96%)[10]

Plantar Foot Pain

Sesamoiditis

HISTORY	MECHANISM OF INJURY	EVALUATION ESSENTIALS
• Patient reports pain on the bottom of the foot specifically at the base of the MTP joint • Patient describes difficulty with flexing or extending great toe	• Increased activity • Repetitive irritation	• Palpation of the sesamoids inferior to the first metatarsal • ROM testing

KEY FINDINGS	DIAGNOSTIC EVIDENCE
• Foot deformities such as pes cavus or lack of fat surrounding sesamoid area • Activities on the ball of the foot will likely be in the history	• MRI and radiographs can help differentiate sesamoid injuries; these include stress fracture (40%), sesamoiditis (30%), acute fracture (10%), osteochondritis (10%), osteoarthritis (5%), and bursitis (5%)[11]

Medial Foot Pain

First Metatarsophalangeal Sprain (Turf Toe)

HISTORY	MECHANISM OF INJURY	EVALUATION ESSENTIALS
• Patient reports pain over the MTP joint • Patient describes difficulty with pushing off the great toe with walking, running, or jumping	• Hyperextension of the great toe acute • Repetitive overuse, typically on synthetic turf	• Palpation of the sesamoids inferior to the first metatarsal • ROM, palpation, and observation • May need referral for imaging depending upon severity

KEY FINDINGS	DIAGNOSTIC EVIDENCE
• Visible swelling at the first MTP joint • Activities in the history include forceful push off on turf or grass	• A grade I to III classification system can be used based on symptoms and clinical findings • Radiographs and MRI can help determine prognosis and determine the need for surgical management[15]

Medial Foot Pain

Hallux Valgus Deformity/Bunion/Exostosis

HISTORY	MECHANISM OF INJURY	EVALUATION ESSENTIALS
• Patient reports pain over the MTP joint • Patient describes increasing pain with walking	• Poorly fitting shoes	• Palpation of the first MTP • ROM and observation

KEY FINDINGS	DIAGNOSTIC EVIDENCE
• Visible deformity at the first MTP • Is often associated with forefoot varus alignment • Flexor and extensor tendons are maligned, creating more stress on the joint • Sesamoiditis and sesamoid fractures can be secondary to hallux valgus	• Hallux abductus angle is measured via radiograph. This measurement is the angle created by the longitudinal axis of the first metatarsal and the hallux. It is considered a reliable indicator of severity of bunions. Over 20 degrees is considered pathologic.[12]

Medial Foot Pain

Tarsal Tunnel Syndrome

HISTORY	MECHANISM OF INJURY	EVALUATION ESSENTIALS
• Patient reports pain along the medial and plantar aspect of the foot • Patient describes burning, numbness, and/or tingling at the foot • Patient complains of increased pain at night	• Any acute trauma to the foot • Tenosynovitis of the medial tendons posterior to the medial malleolus • Previous fracture in the foot or lower leg • Excessive pronation	• Tinel's sign • Lower limb nerve tension test with tibial nerve bias • ROM, palpation, and observation • May need referral for nerve conduction velocity

KEY FINDINGS	DIAGNOSTIC EVIDENCE
• If conditions persists, will see weakness and atrophy following the course of the tibial nerve • His or her pain and/or symptoms will be reproduced with straight leg raise and dorsiflexion and eversion • Patient may also have varicose veins, a tumor on the tibial nerve, or diabetes that may cause the similar symptoms, so thorough history and physical exam is necessary	• Electromyography (EMG) may be useful to examine nerve conduction • MRI may be indicated to identify ganglia or extrinsic masses (83% accuracy) in the tarsal tunnel[14]

Medial Foot Pain

Posterior Tibialis Tendinopathy

HISTORY	MECHANISM OF INJURY	EVALUATION ESSENTIALS
• Patient reports pain along the medial and plantar aspect of the foot • Patient describes aching and fatigue at the medial aspect of the foot • Patient complains of increased swelling with increased activity	• Any acute trauma to the medial ankle • Overuse	• ROM, palpation, and observation • MMT of the posterior tibialis tendon

KEY FINDINGS	DIAGNOSTIC EVIDENCE
• Patient will have pain or an inability to perform a calf raise depending upon severity of the tendinopathy • Pain with posterior tibialis tendon MMT • Most often these patients will present with pes planus and calcaneal eversion foot alignment	• Ultrasound or MRI evaluation of the tendon integrity in persistent cases that do not respond to treatment. MRI has long been considered the gold standard, but ultrasonography has been shown to correlate highly with MR images for tibialis posterior tendinopathy (sensitivity 80%, specificity 90%).[13]

Lateral Foot Pain

Bunionette or Tailor's Bunion

HISTORY	MECHANISM OF INJURY	EVALUATION ESSENTIALS
• Patient reports pain of the 5th MTP joint • Patient describes increasing pain with walking	• Poorly fitting shoes	• Palpation of the fifth MTP • ROM and observation

KEY FINDINGS	DIAGNOSTIC EVIDENCE
• Visible deformity at the fifth MTP • Much less common than hallux valgus • Flexor and extensor tendons are maligned, creating more stress on the joint	• Radiographs can assist with evaluating other deformities and monitoring progression[16]

Lateral Foot Pain

Cuboid Subluxation/Syndrome

HISTORY	MECHANISM OF INJURY	EVALUATION ESSENTIALS
• Patient reports pain upon standing after period of non-weight bearing or with prolonged standing • Patient describes increasing pain with walking along the fourth and fifth metatarsals as well as the cuboid	• Trauma including an inversion mechanism at the ankle	• Palpation of the cuboid • ROM and observation • Calf raise and roll toward your arches

KEY FINDINGS	DIAGNOSTIC EVIDENCE
• May have visible swelling over the cuboid • Tenderness over the cuboid with palpation • Peroneal muscle has stress placed on it by the cuboid during pronation causing pain • Pain is relieved immediately after mobilization	• No diagnostic evidence available

Lateral Foot Pain

Peroneal Tendinopathy

HISTORY	MECHANISM OF INJURY	EVALUATION ESSENTIALS
• Patient reports pain at the lateral or posterolateral ankle and foot • Patient describes increasing pain with activity	• Overuse • Poor footwear and increased training	• Palpation of all the peroneals • ROM, history, and observation • MMT of all the peroneals

KEY FINDINGS	DIAGNOSTIC EVIDENCE
• Most likely have rearfoot varus • Tenderness over the peroneal tendon with palpation • Weakness noted with ankle eversion • Pain is noted with ankle inversion	• Ultrasound or MRI evaluation of the tendon integrity in persistent cases that do not respond to treatment • MRI (sensitivity 84%, specificity 75%)[17] • Ultrasound is advised for a dynamic evaluation of the tendon[18]

Paper Patient: Revisited

In the case of our runner, you should have been able to rule out several conditions secondary to knowing what structures are at the plantar aspect of the foot. Your differential for this case should have been plantar fasciitis, metatarsalgia, or flexor hallucis tendinopathy.

Learning Activities: Practice Case

Use the blank templates provided in the Appendices to write out a differential diagnosis map and clinical findings overview for the case provided below. When working with paper patients, it is tempting to try to jump to "the answer" and come to a diagnosis. However, the visual learning approach to differential diagnosis is designed to help you consider all the possibilities for the information provided. Good luck.

Paper Patient: Foot Pain

History

Rebecca is a 24-year-old college student who states that her feet have been bothering her for about 2 weeks. She exercises regularly and walks on campus daily. She noticed that the tops of her feet were sore after periods of walking. She has been wearing her shoes a bit looser lately. After adjusting her lacing pattern in both shoes, her left foot feels better. Her chief concern is right foot pain. Rebecca describes a throbbing discomfort, and she reports having trouble flexing and extending her toes. She denies a change in her activity volume or intensity. She participated in a dance class last semester with no trouble, and has not had to decrease activity due to her foot pain. She has no numbness or tingling. Pain is a "throbbing" pain; 5/10 at its worst. She states that the foot has had a small amount of swelling in the past 2 weeks. She has no night pain and has not changed her footwear recently.

Physical Exam

The physical exam shows that AROM of the ankle is within normal range, but she reports pain (3/10) at the top of her foot with active plantar flexion. PROM is WNL with normal end feel and also produces pain (3/10) over the dorsal extensor tendons with passive plantar flexion. There is no bony tenderness. Rebecca has a broad area of tenderness and crepitus across the extensor digitorum tendons. Her neurovascular exam is normal. MMT is 5/5 in all planes of movement at the ankle and toes. She has pain (2/10) with resisted ankle dorsiflexion and toe extension.

References

1. Harcourt-Smith WE, Aiello LC. Fossils, feet and the evolution of human bipedal locomotion. *J Anat.* 2004;204(5):403-416.
2. Fernandez WG, Yard EE, Comstock RD. Epidemiology of lower extremity injuries among US high school athletes. *Acad Emerg Med.* 2007;14(7):641-645.
3. National Electronic Injury Surveillance System. *NEISS, the National Electronic Injury Surveillance System: A Tool for Researchers.* Bethesda, MD: US Consumer Product Safety Commission; 2013.
4. Powell JW, Barber-Foss KD. Injury patterns in selected high school sports: A review of the 1995-1997 seasons. *J Athl Train.* 1999;34(3):277-284.
5. Peduto AJ, Read JW. Imaging of ankle tendinopathy and tears. *Top Magn Reson Imaging.* 2010;21(1):25-36.
6. Vanore JV, Christensen JC, Kravitz SR, et al; Clinical Practice Guideline First Metatarasophalangeal Joint Disorders Panel of the American College of Foot and Ankle Surgeons. Diagnosis and treatment of first metatarsophalangeal joint disorders. Section 2: Hallux rigidus. *J Foot Ankle Surg.* 2003;42(3):124-136.
7. Nazarenko A, Beltran LS, Bencardino JT. Imaging evaluation of traumatic ligamentous injuries of the ankle and foot. *Radiol Clin North Am.* 2013;51(3):455-478.
8. Thomas JL, Blitch EL 4th, Chaney DM, et al. Diagnosis and treatment of forefoot disorders. Section 2. Central metatarsalgia. *J Foot Ankle Surg.* 2009;48(2):239-250.
9. Fazal MA, Khan I, Thomas C. Ultrasonography and magnetic resonance imaging in the diagnosis of Morton's neuroma. *J Am Podiatr Med Assoc.* 2012;102(3):184-186.
10. Bolívar YA, Munuera PV, Padillo JP. Relationship between tightness of the posterior muscles of the lower limb and plantar fasciitis. *Foot Ankle Int.* 2013;34(1):42-48.
11. Kindred J, Trubey C, Simons SM. Foot injuries in runners. *Curr Sports Med Rep.* 2011;10(5):249-254.
12. Vanore JV, Christensen JC, Kravitz SR, et al. Diagnosis and treatment of first metatarsophalangeal joint disorders. Section 1: Hallux valgus. *J Foot Ankle Surg.* 2003;42(3):112-123.
13. Premkumar A, Perry MB, Dwyer AJ, et al. Sonography and MR imaging of posterior tibial tendinopathy. *AJR Am J Roentgenol.* 2002;178(1):223-232.
14. Ahmad M, Tsang K, Mackenney PJ, Adedapo AO. Tarsal tunnel syndrome: A literature review. *Foot Ankle Surg.* 2012;18(3):149-152.
15. McCormick JJ, Anderson RB. Turf toe: Anatomy, diagnosis, and treatment. *Sports Health.* 2010;2(6):487-494.
16. Thomas JL, Blitch EL 4th, Chaney DM, et al. Diagnosis and treatment of forefoot disorders. Section 4. Tailor's bunion. *J Foot Ankle Surg.* 2009;48(2):257-263.
17. Park HJ, Cha SD, Kim HS, et al. Reliability of MRI findings of peroneal tendinopathy in patients with lateral chronic ankle instability. *Clin Orthop Surg.* 2010;2(4):237-243.
18. Lee SJ, Jacobson JA, Kim SM, et al. Ultrasound and MRI of the peroneal tendons and associated pathology. *Skeletal Radiol.* 2013;42(9):1191-1200.

3

The Ankle and Lower Leg

Ankle injuries are the most common injury found in a variety of sport activities and athletes who suffer from ankle sprains are more likely to reinjure the same ankle, which can result in disability, chronic pain, or instability. The highest percentage of these injuries occur in sports such as basketball and soccer as they require sudden starts and stops as well as cutting movements. Approximately 25,000 people sprain their ankles on a daily basis.[1] Ankle sprains account for numerous visits to emergency care facilities and significant time loss from sports participation, can cause long-term disability, and have a major impact on health care costs and resources. McGuine and Keene[2] described the impact of ankle sprains in financial terms. Consider that in the United States alone, 4.8 million grade school and 1.7 million high school athletes participate in supervised soccer and basketball programs and, on average, 15% (1 million) of these athletes sustain ankle sprains each year. The costs associated with treating this number of sprains are significant. US Consumer Products Safety Commission estimates place the cost of treating ankle sprains in high school soccer and basketball players (ages 15 to 18 years) at $70 million with indirect costs at $1.1 billion.[3] Given the associated cost, the ability to accurately diagnose ankle sprains and conditions of the ankle and lower leg is of the utmost importance.

The ankle is made up of three general articulations. The talocrural joint is the hinge joint that is formed by the distal tibia and fibula that surround the talus bone. This joint allows for plantar flexion and dorsiflexion of the

Winterstein AP, Clark SV. *The Athletic Trainer's Guide to Differential Diagnosis (pp 35-85).*

foot. The talocrural joint is sometimes called the "true" ankle joint. The distal tibia and fibula are joined at the inferior tibiofibular joint. This joint is held together by the distal syndesmotic membrane. The anterior and posterior tibiofibular ligaments help bind this joint together. The most common motion associated with ankle injury are inversion and eversion. These ankle motions take place below the talus or at the subtalar articulation. Subtalar motion occurs between the talus and the calcaneus. The individual lateral ligaments (anterior talofibular ligament, calcaneofibular ligament, and posterior talofibular ligament) of the ankle tend to be weaker than the stronger medial ligaments (deltoid ligament complex). This ligament arrangement combined with the relative ease of inversion due to the shorter tibia contributes to the frequency of ankle injury.

This chapter provides differential diagnosis maps for the ankle and the lower leg. The ankle and lower leg should be examined together as the lower leg muscles provide both movement and dynamic stability to the ankle joint. In addition, the locations of specific tendons that cross the ankle joint on all four regions of the ankle require careful consideration in the evaluation process. The diagnostic maps for both the ankle and the lower leg have been divided into four regions: anterior, posterior, medial, and lateral. Use of the diagnostic map combined with careful clinical evaluation will provide the user with clear focus as he or she differentiates the ankle and lower leg injuries common to the active patient.

Paper Patient: Ankle Pain in a Recreational Runner

History

Maya is a 40-year-old runner who comes to your clinic complaining of right ankle pain with running. She reports that she runs 3 times per week for 5 to 6 miles every time. She has no mechanism of injury. She points to her lateral ankle as the source of her pain. She runs on the sidewalk or a soft trail, has worn a neutral running shoe, and has never had an issue before. The pain is quite sharp after running and it has been increasing to constant for about the last month. She saw a sports medicine specialist who ordered an MRI that was negative for stress fracture. What it did show was posterior tibialis tendinopathy, although the pain she complains of is not in this location. She noted recently that she has a burning sensation over the lower lateral leg and ankle.

Physical Exam

Her physical exam reveals tenderness to palpation over the peroneal tendon and less so over the posterior tibialis tendon. She has pain with resisted eversion, pain with active inversion and plantar flexion, and no passive motion pain. Her ankle strength was 5/5 in all cardinal planes as well as D1 and D2 pattern motion. She denies pain with active calf raises. Her gait is WNL walking and jogging. Her foot alignment was neutral in standing as well as in subtalar neutral. She had pain with straight leg raise testing on the right at the ankle, and with peroneal nerve bias, the pain the patient feels with running was replicated. Tap test of the peroneal nerve reproduced lateral ankle pain.

Using the information from your clinical exam you will need to ask yourself some questions to guide your clinical decision making:

- What is your differential diagnosis?
- What key findings do you see to help guide your differential?
- What are the possible injuries associated with lateral ankle pain?

Clinical Decisions

Start with a review of the anatomy maps and a thorough consideration of the possible injuries and conditions that are common to the ankle. Use the differential diagnosis maps to guide your thought process and organize the possibilities. The organized synthesis of this information is the essence of clinical decision making.

Anatomy Map: Ankle

ANTERIOR

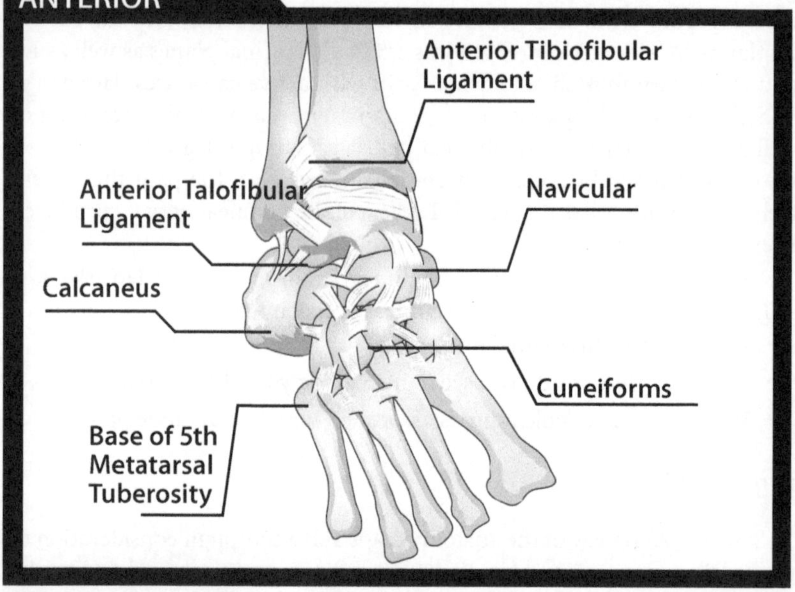

POSTERIOR

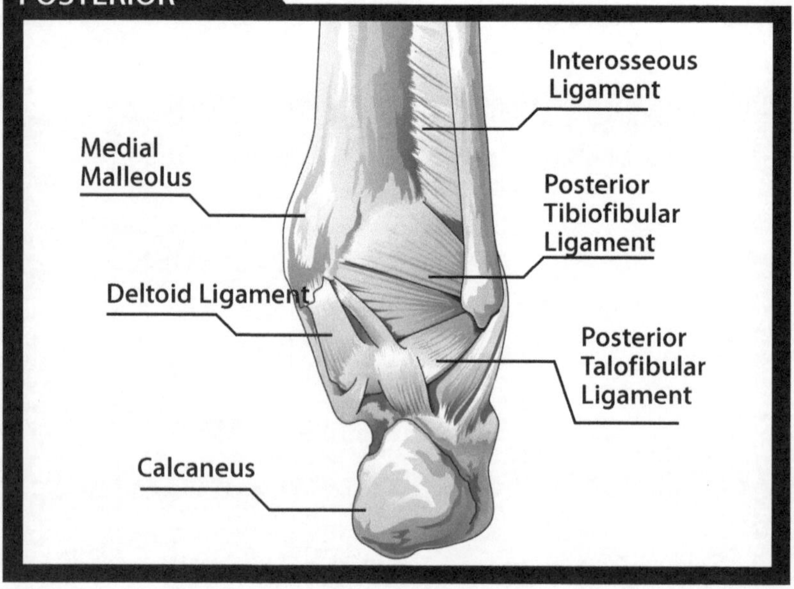

Anatomy Map: Ankle

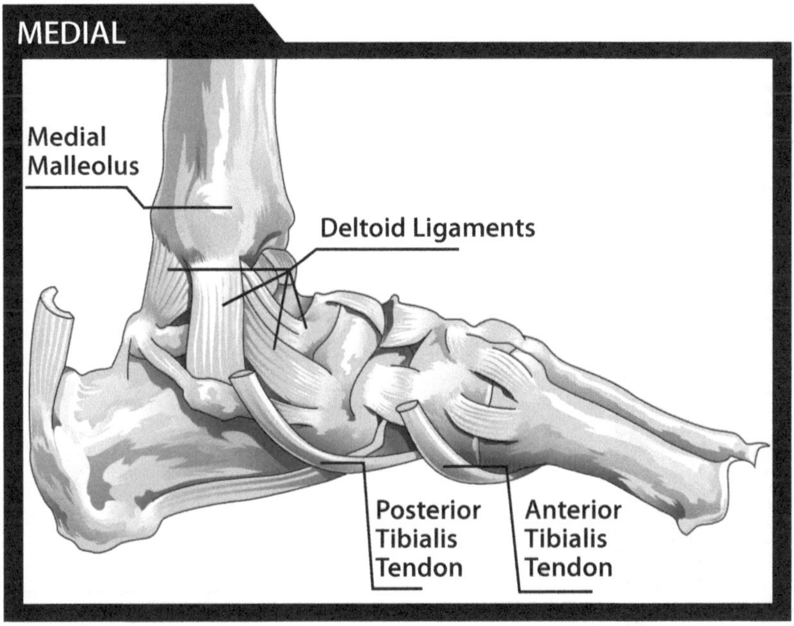

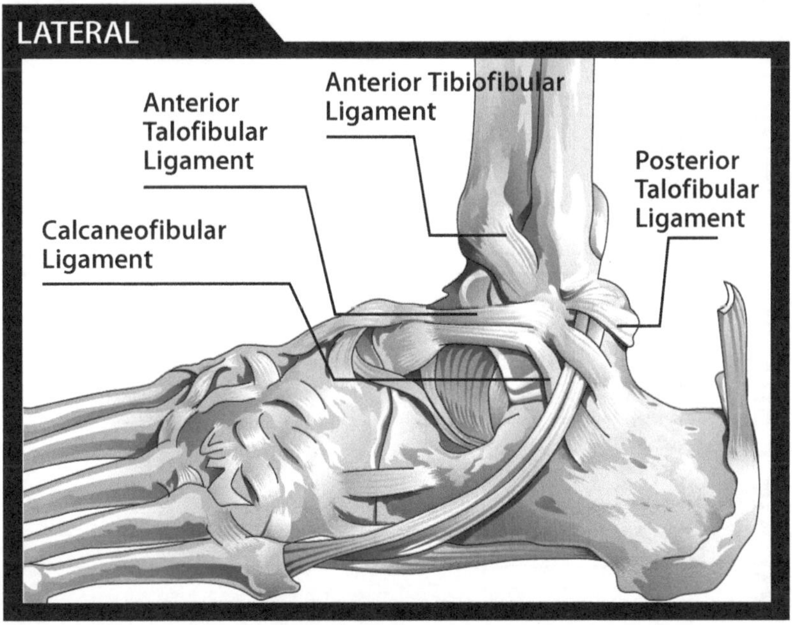

Ankle Pain Map: Region/Soft Tissue Differential Diagnosis

ANTERIOR

- Anterior Impingement (Sinus Tarsi Syndrome)
- Anterior Talofibular Ligament Sprain
- Anterior Tibialis Tendinopathy*
- Anterior Tibiofibular Ligament (Syndesmotic) Sprain
- Extensor Digitorum Longus Tendinopathy
- Extensor Retinaculum Injury

*see Lower Leg map (page 66)

POSTERIOR

- Achilles Tendinopathy*
- Achilles Tendon Rupture*
- Calcaneal/ Retrocalcaneal Bursitis
- Posterior Ankle Impingement
- Posterior Talofibular Ligament Sprain

*see Lower Leg map (pages 67 and 68)

MEDIAL

- Deltoid Ligament Sprain
- Flexor Digitorum Tendinopathy
- Flexor Hallucis Longus Tendinopathy
- Tarsal Tunnel Syndrome (Tibial Nerve Compression)
- Tibialis Posterior Tendinopathy

LATERAL

- Calcaneofibular Ligament Sprain
- Peroneal Tendinopathy
- Subluxing Peroneal Tendons

Ankle Pain

Injuries to Bone/Joint Surfaces

COMMON FRACTURES AND CLASSIFICATIONS

- Distal fibula
- Distal tibia
- Medial/lateral malleolus Weber fracture classification
  - Type A: Vertical medial malleolus compression fracture, horizontal fibula fracture distal to syndesmosis, syndesmosis intact (stable)
  - Type B: Horizontal medial malleolus avulsion fracture, oblique fibula fracture at the level of syndesmosis, syndesmosis sometimes affected (stable-unstable)
  - Type C: Horizontal medial malleolus avulsion fracture, oblique fibula fracture superior to syndesmosis, syndesmosis disrupted (unstable)
- Os trigonum fracture
- Salter-Harris fracture classification for open epiphyses (**SALTR**)
  - Type I: Physis only (**S**eparated)
  - Type II: Physis and metaphysis (**A**bove/proximal to joint)
  - Type III: Physis and epiphysis (**L**ower/distal to joint)
  - Type IV: Physis, metaphysis, and epiphysis (**T**hrough joint)
  - Type V: Compression/crush injury to physis (**R**uined/rammed)
- Talar dome fracture
- Talar osteochondral defect

Clinical Assessment of Ankle Injuries

Anterior Ankle Pain

Anterior Impingement (Sinus Tarsi Syndrome)

HISTORY	MECHANISM OF INJURY	EVALUATION ESSENTIALS
• Patients report chronic pain with dorsiflexion activities • Describes anteromedial, anterocentral, or anterolateral ankle pain • Sport or fitness activities that require repeated dorsiflexion • May have previous history of acute ankle trauma	• Chronic onset • Repeated dorsiflexion	• Assess motion, strength (MMT), and ligamentous stability • Inspection of gait • Perform inversion stress test and anterior drawer • Palpate appropriate bony and ligamentous structures • Assess foot alignment and arch height

KEY FINDINGS	DIAGNOSTIC EVIDENCE
• Tenderness to palpation over the anterior joint line. Anteromedial and anterocentral pain most often secondary to osteophytes off of the tibia or talus. Anterolateral pain is most often soft tissue in nature. • Pain and reproduction of symptoms with dorsiflexion • May develop with overuse and impact activities or secondary to acute trauma	• A positive 5 out of 6 of the following have a sensitivity of 94% and specificity of 75% for predicting anterolateral impingement: chronic ankle pain, anterolateral joint tenderness, recurrent joint swelling, anterolateral pain with forced ankle dorsiflexion and eversion, pain during single-leg squat, and lack of lateral ankle instability.[4]

Anterior Ankle Pain

Anterior Talofibular Ligament Sprain

HISTORY	MECHANISM OF INJURY	EVALUATION ESSENTIALS
• Patient reports acute injury mechanism; often stepping in a hole or landing on another person's foot • A plantar flexion and inversion mechanism of injury (MOI) is described • Pain with weight bearing at distal syndesmosis	• Acute injury • Forced plantar flexion and inversion • Chronic instability may be a secondary issue with repeated injury	• Assess motion and strength • Inspect gait for pain with weight bearing • Perform inversion stress test and anterior drawer • Assess for fracture with bump and compression tests • Balance should be assessed for all chronic instabilities

KEY FINDINGS	DIAGNOSTIC EVIDENCE
• Inspection of gait may reveal avoidance of dorsiflexion • Positive drawer and positive inversion stress tests • Muscle weakness may be noted with acute injury (eg, peroneal weakness) • Persistent instabilities may present with neurological symptoms and must be evaluated accordingly	• Ankle anterior drawer test (sensitivity 100%, specificity 66%)[5] • Clinicians should follow the Ottawa ankle rules with Buffalo modifications to determine the need for radiographic evaluation

Anterior Ankle Pain

Anterior Tibiofibular Ligament Sprain (Syndesmotic)

HISTORY	MECHANISM OF INJURY	EVALUATION ESSENTIALS
• Patient reports acute injury mechanism • Forced dorsiflexion and rotation MOI • Pain with weight bearing at distal syndesmosis	• Rotation of the talus within the ankle mortise • Forced dorsiflexion or plantar flexion (less common) • Common in cutting and pivoting sports	• Assess motion, strength (MMT), and ligamentous stability • Evaluate syndesmosis with dorsiflexion/rotation test and Kleiger's test • Assess distal tibia and fibula for fracture (squeeze test) • Evaluate translation of the distal fibula for stability

KEY FINDINGS	DIAGNOSTIC EVIDENCE
• Inspection of gait may reveal avoidance of dorsiflexion • Tender to palpation over the distal syndesmosis • Positive dorsiflexion rotation test • Mechanism of injury consistent with findings • Pain with motion at extremes of dorsiflexion and plantar flexion	• Radiographs to evaluate ankle mortise and distal syndesmosis (may require stress test radiograph) • Squeeze test (sensitivity 30%, specificity 93.5%) • External rotation test (sensitivity 20%, specificity 84.8%)[6]

Anterior Ankle Pain

Extensor Digitorum Longus Tendinopathy

HISTORY	MECHANISM OF INJURY	EVALUATION ESSENTIALS
• Patient reports pain over anterior region of the ankle • Insidious onset of discomfort • Patient may describe changes in training volume or intensity • Painful gait or pain with repetitive impact activities is reported	• Overuse injury common with repeated eccentric loads • Repetitive dorsiflexion or attenuation of landing forces	• Assess ankle and toe motions for limitation • Check muscle strength through MMT (ankle and toes) • Rule out other injury through joint assessment and neurovascular exam

KEY FINDINGS	DIAGNOSTIC EVIDENCE
• Possible weakness of the extensor digitorum • Tendons are tender to palpation where they cross the anterior ankle • Palpable crepitus may be present • Pain with extension of the toes (second to fifth)	• MRI can be useful to identify edema and inflammatory changes • Ultrasound can detect thickening of the tendon and assess the gliding ability of the tendon through specific ROM[7]

Anterior Ankle Pain

Extensor Retinaculum Injury

HISTORY	MECHANISM OF INJURY	EVALUATION ESSENTIALS
• Patient reports insidious anterior ankle discomfort • May describe changes in training volume or intensity • Reports painful gait or pain with repetitive impact activities • Change in footwear or change in lacing patterns	• Acute or chronic mechanism • Can be injured concomitant to other acute injuries	• Assess ankle motion for limitations • Check muscle strength through MMT (ankle) • Rule out other injury through joint assessment and neurovascular exam

KEY FINDINGS	DIAGNOSTIC EVIDENCE
• Pain with plantar flexion and stretching of the retinacular tissue • Retinacular irritation can be associated with other underlying tendon irritations or secondary to an acute injury following prolonged periods of edema • Often a diagnosis of exclusion • The retinaculum and underlying tendons can be irritated secondary to tightness along the lacing patterns of the shoe	• No diagnostic evidence available

Posterior Ankle Pain

Calcaneal/Retrocalcaneal Bursitis

HISTORY	MECHANISM OF INJURY	EVALUATION ESSENTIALS
• Patient reports an insidious onset of discomfort • Patient may describe changes in training volume or intensity • Painful gait with pain at push off (into plantar flexion) • May describe a change in footwear with rubbing at the calcaneus	• Overuse injury common with repeated eccentric loads • Repetitive resisted plantar flexion or attenuation of landing forces • Patient may report recent change in footwear or ill-fitting footwear	• Assess AROM and PROM at the ankle • Evaluate strength (MMT) for gastrocnemius and soleus • Inspection may reveal visible area of swelling at the insertion of the Achilles tendon • Palpation or pinching maneuver between tendon and bone

KEY FINDINGS	DIAGNOSTIC EVIDENCE
• Must be differentiated from Achilles tendinopathy and also differentiated from the subcutaneous bursa on the most posterior aspect of calcaneus. • Pain elicited with pinching of the retrocalcaneal bursa	• MRI: A bursa larger than 1 mm anteroposteriorly, 11 mm horizontally, or 7 mm craniocaudally is abnormal[8]

Posterior Ankle Pain

Posterior Ankle Impingement

HISTORY	MECHANISM OF INJURY	EVALUATION ESSENTIALS
• Patient may report chronic or recurrent posterior ankle pain • Pain exacerbated by forceful plantar flexion and push off activities (eg, dancing, kicking, downhill running) • Painful gait with pain at push off (into plantar flexion)	• Repetitive forced plantar flexion • Acute mechanisms are also possible	• Assess motion and strength (MMT) • Inspection of gait may reveal avoidance of plantar flexion • Rule out other injury through joint assessment (ligamentous stability) and neurovascular exam

KEY FINDINGS	DIAGNOSTIC EVIDENCE
• Diagnostic imaging may reveal pathology of the os trigonum (posterior process of the talus) • Most often diagnosed based on clinical history and physical exam • MRI may also reveal pathology of the flexor hallicus longus tendinopathy, osteochondritis, subtalar joint disease, and fractures	• Sensitivity and specificity of radiographs and MRI have not been reported in the literature, but are considered standard of care for evaluating bony and soft tissue structures[9]

Posterior Ankle Pain

Posterior Talofibular Ligament Sprain

HISTORY	MECHANISM OF INJURY	EVALUATION ESSENTIALS
• Patient reports an acute injury possible dislocation or extreme dorsiflexion • Acute onset injury • Pain with dorsiflexion • May not be able to ambulate	• Acute MOI • Dorsiflexion and rotation MOI possible dislocation	• Assess motion, strength (MMT), and ligamentous stability • Inspect gait to assess weight bearing • Perform inversion, anterior drawer, and dorsiflexion ER tests. • Palpate bony and soft tissue structures • Compression, squeeze, and bump tests

KEY FINDINGS	DIAGNOSTIC EVIDENCE
• The posterior talofibular ligament is rarely injured in isolation. It is usually torn in association with other ligament injuries (anterior talofibular ligament and calcaneofibular ligament) or with dislocation of the talus. • Fibers of the posterior talofibular ligament are oriented horizontally and under tension in extreme dorsiflexion	• Clinicians should follow the Ottawa ankle rules with Buffalo modifications to determine the need for radiographic evaluation[10]

Medial Ankle Pain

Deltoid Ligament Sprain

HISTORY

- Patient reports acute injury mechanism
- Describes forced eversion; often an opposing player lands or rolls up on lateral lower leg
- Pain with weight bearing and may describe instability

MECHANISM OF INJURY

- Planted foot with pronation-abduction or planted foot with forced rotation
- Common in cutting and pivoting sports
- Similar mechanism as the syndesmotic sprain

EVALUATION ESSENTIALS

- Assess motion, strength, and ligamentous stability
- Evaluate deltoid ligament and syndesmosis with dorsiflexion/rotation and Kleiger's tests
- Compression and bump tests for fracture

KEY FINDINGS

- Inspection of gait may reveal avoidance of dorsiflexion
- Full ruptures of the deltoid ligaments are often associated with fractures
- Significant forces are required to injure the strong deltoid. The injury often continues through the syndesmosis.

DIAGNOSTIC EVIDENCE

- Clinicians should follow the Ottawa ankle rules with Buffalo modifications to determine the need for radiographic evaluation
- External rotation test (sensitivity 20%, specificity 84.8%)[6]

Medial Ankle Pain

Flexor Digitorum Tendinopathy

HISTORY	MECHANISM OF INJURY	EVALUATION ESSENTIALS
• Patient reports pain over medial region of the ankle behind medial malleolus • Insidious onset of discomfort • Patient may describe changes in training volume or intensity • May report discomfort with flexion of toes (second to fifth)	• Overuse injury common with repeated eccentric loads • May present following an ankle sprain due to lack of motion or if rehabilitation exercises are too aggressive • Common secondary to chronic ankle instability	• Assess ankle motion • Check muscle strength through MMT (ankle) • Palpate distal tendons on the distal plantar surface of foot (toes 2 to 5) • Rule out other injury through joint assessment and neurovascular exam

KEY FINDINGS	DIAGNOSTIC EVIDENCE
• Possible weakness and pain with resisted toe flexion (second to fifth) and ankle plantar flexion • Tendon is tender to palpation where it crosses the medial ankle • Palpable crepitus may be present • Pes planus foot and rearfoot pronation may be predisposing factors • Activities that require patients to go up on the toes may contribute to flexor digitorum longus tendinopathy	• MRI can be useful to identify edema and inflammatory changes • Ultrasound can detect thickening of the tendon and assess the gliding ability of the tendon through specific ROM[7]

Medial Ankle Pain

Flexor Hallucis Longus Tendinopathy

HISTORY	MECHANISM OF INJURY	EVALUATION ESSENTIALS
• Patient reports pain over medial region of the ankle behind medial malleolus • Insidious onset of discomfort • Patient may describe changes in training volume or intensity • May report discomfort with flexion of the great toe	• Overuse injury common with repeated eccentric loads • May present following an ankle sprain due to lack of motion or if rehabilitation exercises are too aggressive • Common secondary to chronic ankle instability	• Assess ankle motion • Check muscle strength through MMT (ankle) • Palpate distal tendon on the plantar surface of the great toe • Rule out other injury through joint assessment and neurovascular exam

KEY FINDINGS	DIAGNOSTIC EVIDENCE
• Possible weakness and pain with resisted great toe flexion and ankle plantar flexion • Tendon is tender to palpation where it crosses the medial ankle • Palpable crepitus may be present • Pes planus foot and rearfoot pronation may be predisposing factors • Activities that require patients to go up on the toes may contribute to FHL tendinopathy	• MRI can be useful to identify edema and inflammatory changes • Ultrasound can detect thickening of the tendon and assess the gliding ability of the tendon through specific ROM[7]

Medial Ankle Pain

Tarsal Tunnel Syndrome (Tibial Nerve Compression)

HISTORY	MECHANISM OF INJURY	EVALUATION ESSENTIALS
• Patients note pain and foot numbness • May describe pain radiating along the plantar side of the foot and up into the gastrocnemius • Pain identified with extremes of dorsiflexion	• Chronic onset • Footwear compression may be implicated • May be caused by lipoma, ganglia, or neoplasms in the tarsal tunnel • Accessory flexor digitorum longus muscle can cause compression in tarsal tunnel	• Assess motion, strength, and ligamentous stability • Evaluation of medial lower leg tendinopathies is essential for differential diagnosis • Tinel test over tarsal tunnel • Passive eversion-external rotation test • Lower quarter neurological assessment

KEY FINDINGS	DIAGNOSTIC EVIDENCE
• Presence of rearfoot valgus can be a predisposing factor • Tibial nerve tension is increased by eversion and dorsiflexion of the foot • Tinel sign behind the medial malleolus is often positive • Compressing the tibial nerve for a period of 30 seconds may reproduce symptoms	• EMG may be useful to examine nerve conduction • MRI may be indicated to identify ganglia or extrinsic masses (83% accuracy) in the tarsal tunnel[11]

Medial Ankle Pain

Tibialis Posterior Tendinopathy

HISTORY	MECHANISM OF INJURY	EVALUATION ESSENTIALS
• Patient reports pain over medial region of the ankle behind medial malleolus • Insidious onset of discomfort • Patient may describe changes in training volume or intensity • May report discomfort into the foot at navicular tubercle	• Overuse injury common with repeated eccentric loads • May present following an ankle sprain due to lack of motion or if rehabilitation exercises are too aggressive • Common secondary to chronic ankle instability	• Assess ankle motion • Check muscle strength through MMT (ankle) • Palpate distal tendon behind malleolus to the insertion at navicular tubercle • Rule out other injury through joint assessment and neurovascular exam

KEY FINDINGS	DIAGNOSTIC EVIDENCE
• Possible weakness and pain with resisted inversion and plantar flexion • Tendons are tender to palpation where they cross the medial ankle • Palpable crepitus may be present • Pes planus foot and rearfoot pronation may be predisposing factors • Stress reaction must be considered with persistent pain at insertion of tibialis posterior	• Ultrasound or MRI evaluation of the tendon integrity in persistent cases that do not respond to treatment. MRI has long been considered the gold standard, but ultrasonography has been shown to correlate highly with MR images for tibialis posterior tendinopathy (sensitivity 80%, specificity 90%).[12]

Lateral Ankle Pain

Calcaneofibular Ligament Sprain

HISTORY	MECHANISM OF INJURY	EVALUATION ESSENTIALS
• Patient reports acute injury mechanism • Describes forced inversion • Patient describes pain with weight bearing • May describe instability	• Acute Injury • Subtalar inversion • Chronic instability may be a secondary issue with repeated injury	• Assess motion and strength • Inspect gait for pain with weight bearing • Evaluate ligamentous integrity with inversion stress test • Assess for fracture with bump and compression tests

KEY FINDINGS	DIAGNOSTIC EVIDENCE
• Tender to palpation over the calcaneofibular ligament • Pain and instability with inversion stress test • Mechanism of injury consistent with findings	• Clinicians should follow the Ottawa ankle rules with Buffalo modifications to determine the need for radiographic evaluation • Inversion stress test validity and reliability has not been reported in the literature. A positive test for laxity is often considered to be a side to side difference of at least 10 degrees.[10]

Lateral Ankle Pain

Peroneal Tendinopathy

HISTORY	MECHANISM OF INJURY	EVALUATION ESSENTIALS
• Patient reports pain over lateral region of the ankle • Insidious onset of discomfort • Patient may describe changes in training volume or intensity	• Overuse injury common with repeated eccentric loads • Common secondary to ankle sprain due to lack of motion or too aggressive strength exercises • Common secondary to chronic ankle instability	• Assess ankle motion • Check muscle strength through MMT (ankle) • Rule out other injury through joint assessment and neurovascular exam • Take special care to evaluate peroneus brevis insertion at base of fifth metatarsal

KEY FINDINGS	DIAGNOSTIC EVIDENCE
• Possible weakness of the peroneal muscle group; pain with resisted eversion • Tendons are tender to palpation where they cross the lateral ankle • Palpable crepitus may be present • Balance test may reveal chronic instability	• Ultrasound or MRI evaluation of the tendon integrity in persistent cases that do not respond to treatment • MRI (sensitivity 84%, specificity 75%)[13] • Ultrasound is advised for a dynamic evaluation of the tendon[14]

Lateral Ankle Pain

Subluxing Peroneal Tendons

HISTORY	MECHANISM OF INJURY	EVALUATION ESSENTIALS
• Patient may report a specific acute inversion ankle injury • Can also be a chronic manifestation of repeated ankle sprains • Pain identified with functional ankle activities	• Acute inversion MOI • Tearing of lateral retinaculum • Chronic onset secondary to ankle instability	• Assess ankle motion • Check muscle strength through MMT (ankle) • Observe for subluxing of peroneals at the end range of eversion • Rule out other injury through joint assessment and neurovascular exam

KEY FINDINGS	DIAGNOSTIC EVIDENCE
• Physical exam may be normal until subluxation of tendons from the fibular groove occurs • Moderate to severe pain with subluxation • Pes cavus foot may be a predisposing factor creating increased tension on the peroneal tendons	• Ultrasonography (sensitivity 100%, specificity 90%) or MRI (sensitivity 23%, specificity 100%) evaluation of the tendon integrity in persistent cases that do not respond to treatment[15]

Paper Patient—Ankle: Revisited

In the case of Maya, our 40-year-old runner, you should have been able to rule out several conditions secondary to knowing what structures are at the lateral ankle. Your differential for her case should have been peroneal tendinopathy versus peroneal nerve tension.

Paper Patient: Lower Leg Pain in a Marathon Runner

History

Karen is a 47-year-old runner who complains of right side posterior lower leg pain. She reports that she had completed a half marathon at the end of November and was disappointed with her time. She decided in January to increase her running speed while running on the treadmill. She normally runs outside but in the winter will run on the treadmill if it is icy outside. The winter has been quite icy so she has been running almost exclusively on the treadmill. She increased her speed by 0.5 to 1.0 miles per hour and ran for 3 to 4 miles at a time. After starting this 3 weeks ago, she had a morning where she noted limping that did not subside secondary to pain. She decided to stop running because she was limping during the day. She has been walking on the treadmill at a brisk pace with grade and this does not hurt. She notes having stiffness in the ankle every morning when she gets up to take her first steps.

Physical Exam

Your physical exam found tenderness to palpation over the distal Achilles tendon on the right. The patient had pain with active plantar flexion during a calf raise. The patient feels stiffness with passive dorsiflexion in a long seated position. The patient had decreased strength of the hip external rotators and core with MMT.

Negative ligamentous testing at the ankle, it is noted that the patient has mild laxity that is bilateral. Retrocalcaneal bursal squeeze test was negative. No deformity is observed and there is mild navicular drop, mild calcaneal eversion, and genu varum in standing.

Clinical Decisions

Using the information from your clinical exam you will need to ask yourself some questions to guide your clinical decision making:

- What is your differential diagnosis?
- What key findings do you see to help guide your differential?
- What are the possible injuries associated with lower leg and ankle pain?

Consider Karen's case by reviewing the anatomy maps and given thorough consideration to the possible injuries and conditions that are common to the lower leg. Use the differential diagnosis maps to guide your thought process and organize the possibilities. The organized synthesis of this information is the essence of clinical decision making. We will revisit this case at the end of the chapter.

Anatomy Map: Lower Leg

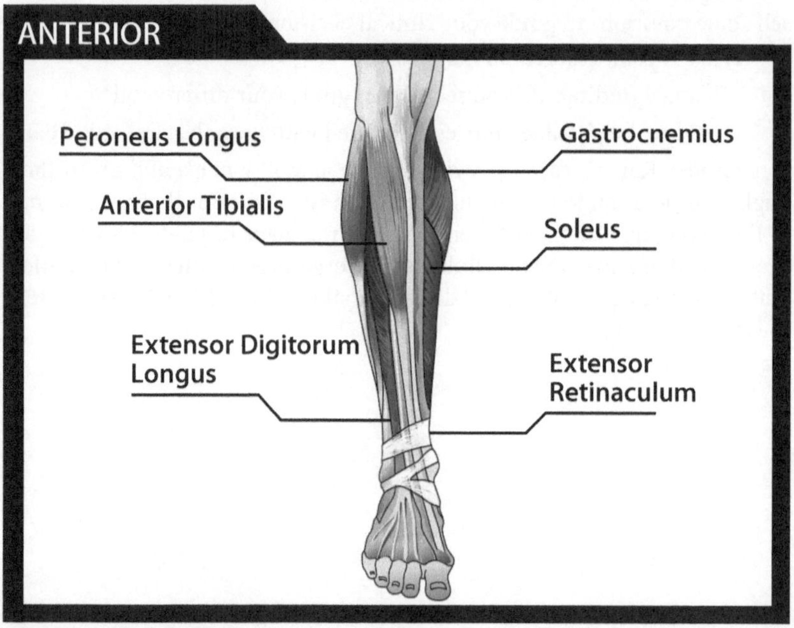

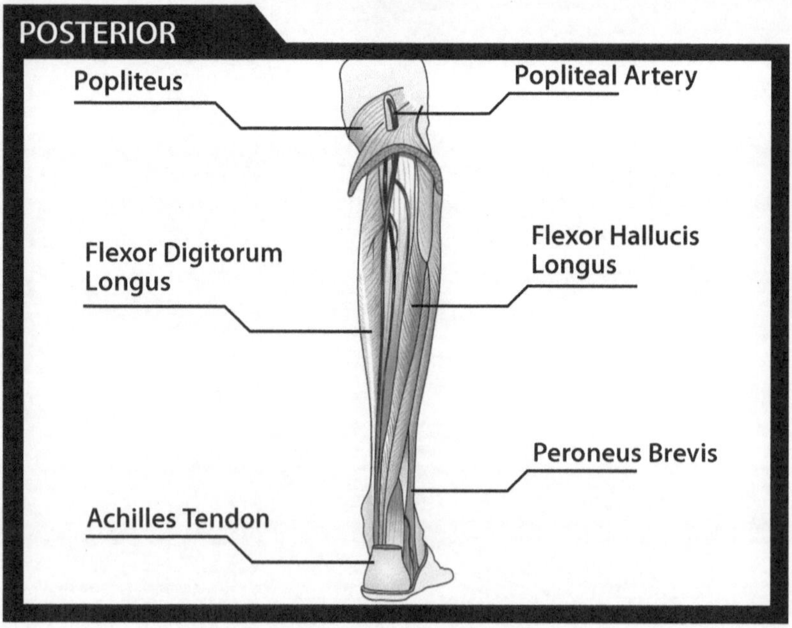

Anatomy Map: Lower Leg

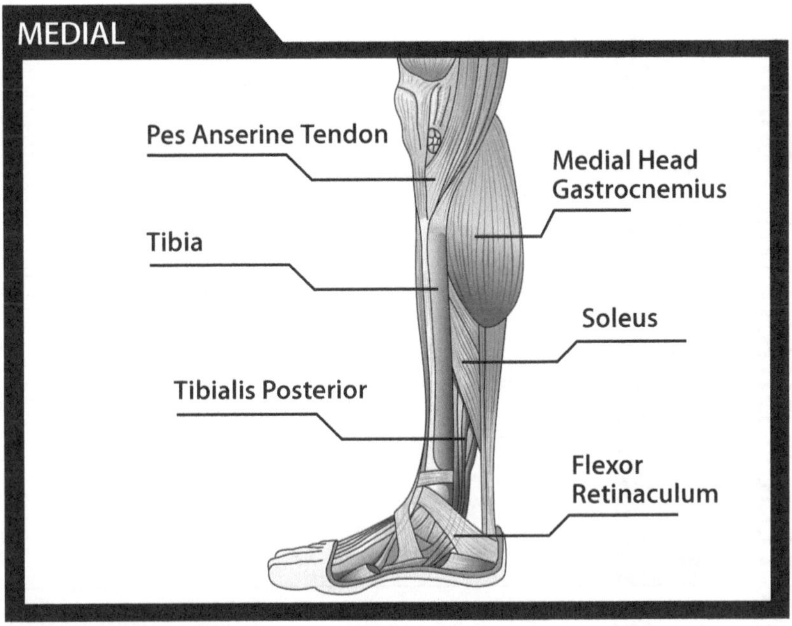

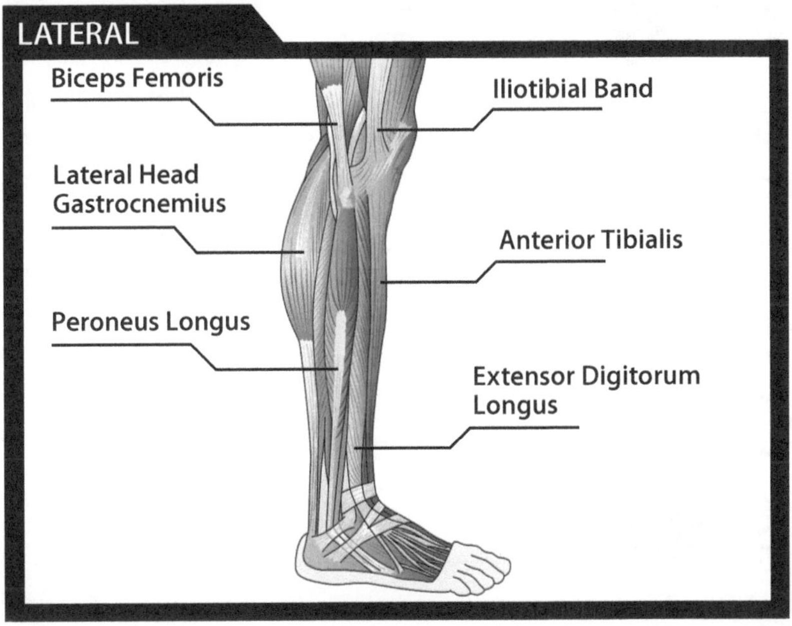

Lower Leg Map: Region/Soft Tissue Differential Diagnosis

ANTERIOR

- Anterior Compartment Syndrome
- Tibialis Anterior Strain
- Anterior Tibialis Tendinopathy

POSTERIOR

- Achilles Tendinopathy
- Achilles Tendon Rupture
- Deep Posterior Compartment Syndrome
- Deep Vein Thrombosis (DVT)
- Gastrocnemius Strain
- Gastrocnemius Tendinopathy
- Popliteus Strain
- Posterior Superficial Compartment Syndrome
- Soleus Strain
- Soleus Tendinopathy

MEDIAL

- Flexor Digitorum Strain
- Flexor Hallicus Tendinopathy*
- Medial Tibial Stress Syndrome
- Tibialis Posterior Strain
- Tibialis Posterior Tendinopathy*

**See Ankle Map (pages 52 and 54)*

LATERAL

- Lateral Compartment Syndrome
- Peroneal Neuropathy
- Peroneal Strain
- Peroneal Tendinopathy*

**See Ankle Map (page 56)*

Lower Leg Pain

Injuries to Bone/Joint Surfaces

COMMON FRACTURES

- Fibula stress fracture
- Fibular head
- Pilon fracture
- Proximal fibular shaft (Maissoneuve)
- Tib-fib fracture
- Segund fracture
- Tibial fractures
    - Plateau (see knee injuries)
    - Shaft
    - Plafond (see ankle injuries)
- Tibial stress fracture

Note: Stress fractures can result from mechanical loading factors and/or metabolic issues leading to insufficiency in bone health. Careful consideration must be given to patient history, activity level, and bone health. Stress fractures to the tibia are common and must be refered for appropriate follow up.

Clinical Assessment of Lower Leg Injuries

Anterior Lower Leg Pain

Anterior Compartment Syndrome

HISTORY	MECHANISM OF INJURY	EVALUATION ESSENTIALS
• Patient reports tightness in lower leg, and deep aching pain • Chronic or acute onset • Pain identified with activity that subsides when activity stops	• Acute occurs due to a direct trauma • Chronic usually occurs with running and jumping activities at a certain point during activity • Acute exertional compartment syndrome may involve minimal to moderate trauma	• Assess tenderness to palpation • Inspect lower leg for distal pulse • Referral for pressure measurement • Evaluate muscle strength

KEY FINDINGS	DIAGNOSTIC EVIDENCE
• History will correlate to the physical exam • Anterior is the most common • The patient will have pain, swelling, and neurovascular symptoms due to the structures in the anterior compartment	• Acute compartment intra-compartmental pressure monitoring (sensitivity 94%, specificity 98%)[16] • MRI for chronic compartment syndrome (sensitivity 96%, specificity 87%)[17]

Anterior Lower Leg Pain

Tibialis Anterior Strain

HISTORY	MECHANISM OF INJURY	EVALUATION ESSENTIALS
• Patient reports pain in the anterior lower leg • Acute onset • Pain identified with specific activity and then with activities of daily life (ADLs)	• Forceful eccentric contraction	• Assess MMT for inversion with dorsiflexion • Inspect muscle and tendon

KEY FINDINGS	DIAGNOSTIC EVIDENCE
• The patient will have pain with inversion and dorsiflexion • The patient will have pain in the anterior lower leg	• No diagnostic evidence available

Anterior Ankle Pain

Anterior Tibialis Tendinopathy

HISTORY	MECHANISM OF INJURY	EVALUATION ESSENTIALS
• Patient reports pain over anterior region of the ankle • Insidious onset of discomfort • Patient may describe changes in training volume or intensity • Painful gait or pain with repetitive impact activities is reported	• Overuse injury common with repeated eccentric loads • Repetitive dorsiflexion or attenuation of landing forces	• Assess ankle motion for limitations • Check muscle strength through MMT (ankle) • Rule out other injury through joint assessment and neurovascular exam

KEY FINDINGS	DIAGNOSTIC EVIDENCE
• Possible weakness of the anterior tibialis tendon • Tendon is tender to palpation where it crosses the anterior ankle; may be tender at the insertion on the navicular bone of the foot • Palpable crepitus may be present • Pain with ankle dorsiflexion at tendon; may have associated anterior shin pain	• MRI can be useful to identify edema and inflammatory changes • Ultrasound can detect thickening of the tendon and assess the gliding ability of the tendon through specific ROM[7]

Posterior Lower Leg Pain

Achilles Tendinopathy

HISTORY

- Patient reports an insidious onset of discomfort
- Patient may describe changes in training volume or intensity
- Painful gait and pain at push off (into plantar flexion)
- May describe a squeaky sensation

MECHANISM OF INJURY

- Overuse injury common with repeated eccentric loads
- Repetitive resisted plantar flexion or attenuation of landing forces
- May have an acute rapid onset (tendinitis) or chronic onset secondary to tissue changes

EVALUATION ESSENTIALS

- Assess motion (active and passive) at the ankle
- Evaluate strength (MMT) for gastrocnemius and soleus
- Inspection may reveal visible nodules or inflammation at distal tendon
- Palpate to determine pain and crepitus

KEY FINDINGS

- Palpable crepitus or presence of a nodule at distal tendon
- Pain in dorsiflexion due to stretch on tendon
- History consistent with onset of symptoms

DIAGNOSTIC EVIDENCE

- Chronic tendinosis may present with a concomitant tear in the tendon tissue
- Ultrasound evaluation of the tendon integrity in persistent cases that do not respond to treatment (sensitivity 80%, 49%)
- MRI imaging of the Achilles tendon for tendinopathy (sensitivity 95%, specificity 50%)[18]

Posterior Lower Leg Pain

Achilles Tendon Rupture

HISTORY	MECHANISM OF INJURY	EVALUATION ESSENTIALS
• Patient reports an acute episode • May describe a sensation of being "kicked in the calf" • Commonly describe an audible "pop" or popping sensation • Describes a history of Achilles tendinopathy	• Forced plantar flexion • High velocity eccentric load	• Inspect the contour of the gastrocnemius and Achilles tendon • Palpate for pain, swelling, and palpable defect • Assess ankle motion (active and passive) • Check muscle strength through MMT (ankle) • Perform a Thompson test • Neurovascular exam must be completed to assess distal pulse

KEY FINDINGS	DIAGNOSTIC EVIDENCE
• More common in middle aged "weekend warrior" participants and more common in male participants • Weak plantar flexion may still be possible due to other musculature • Pain with active and passive motions; use caution as passive doriflexion places stress on injury site • Palpable defect may be present but can be difficult to palpate secondary to swelling	• Most Achilles ruptures are evident; however, MRI or ultrasound evaluation of the tendon integrity may be used to assess extent of the tear • Thompson test (sensitivity 96%, specificity 93%)[19]

Posterior Lower Leg Pain

Posterior Deep Compartment Syndrome

HISTORY	MECHANISM OF INJURY	EVALUATION ESSENTIALS
• Patient reports tightness in lower leg, and deep aching pain • Chronic or acute onset • Pain identified with activity that subsides when activity stops	• Acute occurs due to a direct trauma • Chronic usually occurs with running and jumping activities at a certain point and in time during the activity • Acute exertional is not due to trauma; it can involve minimal to moderate trauma	• Assess tenderness to palpation • Inspect lower leg for distal pulse • Referral for pressure measurement • Evaluate muscle strength

KEY FINDINGS	DIAGNOSTIC EVIDENCE
• Pain will be posterior • History will correlate to the physical exam • The patient will have pain, swelling, and neurovascular symptoms due to the structures in the posterior compartment	• Acute compartment intra-compartmental pressure monitoring (sensitivity 94%, specificity 98%)[16] • MRI for chronic compartment syndrome (sensitivity 96%, specificity 87%)[17]

Posterior Lower Leg Pain

Deep Vein Thrombosis

HISTORY	MECHANISM OF INJURY	EVALUATION ESSENTIALS
• Patient reports mild to severe pain, swelling, and color change in the posterior lower leg • Acute onset • Pain identified with movement	• In the athletic population, it is typically a post surgical patient with prolonged rest or immobilization • History of DVT, prolonged sitting or bed rest, obesity, smoking, heart failure, pregnancy, cancer, or taking HRT or birth control medication	• Homan's sign • Inspect for erythema and swelling in the posterior lower leg and possibly the ankle • Palpate for warmth • Ultrasonography, venography, blood testing, and either MRI or CT are used for definitive diagnosis

KEY FINDINGS	DIAGNOSTIC EVIDENCE
• The patient will have pain in the posterior leg or behind the knee • History and physical exam will correlate • If patient complains of shortness of breath as well need to consider pulmonary embolism • May occur in other areas post surgically • History must inquire recent travel and prolonged sitting (eg, car rides or plane trips)	• D-dimer blood test (sensitivity 85% to 96%, specificity 71% to 99%) • Compression ultrasonography (sensitivity 94%, specificity 98%) • CT (sensitivity 96%, specificity 95%) • MRI (sensitivity 92%, specificity 94.8%)[20]

Posterior Lower Leg Pain

Gastrocnemius Strain

HISTORY	MECHANISM OF INJURY	EVALUATION ESSENTIALS
• Patient reports pain in the posterior lower leg • Acute onset • Pain identified with specific activity and then with ADLs	• Forceful eccentric contraction • Quick stops and starts • Strains are more common in the medial head of the gastrocnemius at or near the musculo-tendinous junction	• Assess MMT for knee flexion and plantar flexion of the foot • Inspect muscle and tendon

KEY FINDINGS	DIAGNOSTIC EVIDENCE
• The patient may have pain with either knee flexion, plantar flexion of the foot, or combination of both • The patient will have pain in the posterior lower leg and possibly swelling • History and physical exam will correlate	• Diagnostic ultrasound is considered less sensitive for detecting calf strains than MRI and is user dependent[21]

Posterior Lower Leg Pain

Gastrocnemius Tendinopathy

HISTORY	MECHANISM OF INJURY	EVALUATION ESSENTIALS
• Patient reports pain and tightness in the back of the knee • Acute or chronic onset	• This is usually an overuse injury • Excessive hill running or increase in mileage	• Inspect posterior lower leg for swelling • Palpable for tenderness of the gastrocnemius at the site of injury • Evaluate muscle strength of the gastrocnemius

KEY FINDINGS	DIAGNOSTIC EVIDENCE
• There will be pain with MMT of the gastrocnemius • The history and physical exam will correlate	• Diagnostic evidence for tendinopathy of the calf focuses on the Achilles tendon complex • Ultrasound evaluation of the tendon integrity in persistent cases that do not respond to treatment (sensitivity 80%, specificity 49%) • MRI imaging of the Achilles tendon for tendinopathy (sensitivity 95%, specificity 50%)[17]

Posterior Lower Leg Pain

Popliteus Strain

HISTORY	MECHANISM OF INJURY	EVALUATION ESSENTIALS
• Patient reports pain in the posterolateral proximal leg • Acute onset • Pain identified with trying to run	• Anteromedial force to the posterior leg causing tibial external rotation	• Assess MMT for popliteus muscle • Garrick's test is positive: pain with resisted external rotation of the tibia • Inspect muscle and tendon for edema

KEY FINDINGS	DIAGNOSTIC EVIDENCE
• The patient will have pain with passive knee flexion and internal rotation • The patient will have pain in the posterolateral leg or behind the knee • History and physical exam will correlate • These injuries are uncommon	• MRI can be used to assess soft tissue injury[22]

Lower Leg Pain

Posterior Superficial Compartment Syndrome

HISTORY

- Patient reports tightness in lower leg and deep aching pain
- Chronic or acute onset
- Pain identified with activity that subsides when activity stops

MECHANISM OF INJURY

- Acute occurs due a direct trauma
- Chronic usually occurs with running and jumping activities at a certain point and in time during the activity
- Acute exertional is not due to trauma; it can involve minimal to moderate trauma

EVALUATION ESSENTIALS

- Assess tenderness to palpation
- Inspect lower leg for distal pulse
- Referral for pressure measurement
- Evaluate muscle strength

KEY FINDINGS

- Pain will be posterior
- The patient will have pain and swelling
- History will correlate to the physical exam

DIAGNOSTIC EVIDENCE

- Acute compartment intra-compartmental pressure monitoring (sensitivity 94%, specificity 98%)[16]
- MRI for chronic compartment syndrome (sensitivity 96%, specificity 87%)[17]

Lower Leg Pain

Soleus Strain

HISTORY	MECHANISM OF INJURY	EVALUATION ESSENTIALS
• Patient reports pain in the posterior lower leg • Acute onset • Pain identified with specific activity and then with ADLs	• Forceful eccentric contraction	• Assess MMT for plantar flexion of the foot with knee flexed • Inspect muscle and tendon

KEY FINDINGS	DIAGNOSTIC EVIDENCE
• The patient will have pain with plantar flexion of the foot with knee flexed • The patient will have pain in the posterior lower leg • History and physical exam will correlate	• Diagnostic ultrasound is considered less sensitive for detecting calf strains than MRI and is user dependent[21]

Posterior Lower Leg Pain

Soleus Tendinopathy

HISTORY	MECHANISM OF INJURY	EVALUATION ESSENTIALS
• Patient reports pain and tightness in the back of the knee below the joint • Acute or chronic onset	• This is usually an overuse injury • Excessive hill running or increase in mileage	• Inspect posterior lower leg for swelling • Palpable for tenderness of the soleus at the site of injury • Evaluate muscle strength of the soleus

KEY FINDINGS	DIAGNOSTIC EVIDENCE
• There will be pain with MMT of the soleus • The history and physical exam will correlate	• Diagnostic evidence for tendinopathy of the calf focuses on the Achilles tendon complex • Ultrasound evaluation of the tendon integrity in persistent cases that do not respond to treatment (sensitivity 80%, specificity 49%) • MRI imaging of the Achilles tendon for tendinopathy (sensitivity 95%, specificity 50%)[18]

Medial Lower Leg Pain

Flexor Digitorum Strain

HISTORY	MECHANISM OF INJURY	EVALUATION ESSENTIALS
• Patient reports pain in the medial lower leg • Acute onset • Pain identified with specific activity and with ADLs	• Forceful eccentric contraction	• Assess MMT plantar flexion and inversion and toe flexion • Inspect muscle and tendon

KEY FINDINGS	DIAGNOSTIC EVIDENCE
• The patient will have pain with plantar flexion, flexion of the toes, and inversion of the foot • The patient will have pain in the medial lower leg • History and physical exam will correlate	• No diagnostic evidence available

Medial Lower Leg Pain

Medial Tibial Stress Syndrome

HISTORY	MECHANISM OF INJURY	EVALUATION ESSENTIALS
• Patient reports shin pain • Chronic onset • Pain identified with exercise and then sometimes with activities of daily living (ADLs) • Patient may also report pain before or after exercise	• Repetitive micro trauma • Other contributing factors include muscle weakness, poor shoes, training errors, and biomechanical issues of the foot	• Bump and compression testing of the lower leg • Assess tenderness along the medial tibial shaft • Inspect for swelling • Evaluate muscle strength of lower leg muscles both anterior and posterior

KEY FINDINGS	DIAGNOSTIC EVIDENCE
• The patient can have pain before, during, or after activity in any combination • The bump and compression tests will be negative • The patient will have palpable tenderness along the medial tibial shaft	• MRI (sensitivity 79% to 88%, specificity 33% to 100%) • Proven risk factors: pronation, female sex, increased internal and external hip ranges of motion, higher BMI, previous history of MTSS, and leaner calf girth[22]

Medial Lower Leg Pain

Tibialis Posterior Strain

HISTORY	MECHANISM OF INJURY	EVALUATION ESSENTIALS
• Patient reports pain in the medial lower leg • Acute onset • Pain identified with specific activity and then with ADLs	• Forceful eccentric contraction	• Assess MMT plantar flexion and inversion • Inspect muscle and tendon

KEY FINDINGS	DIAGNOSTIC EVIDENCE
• The patient will have pain with plantar flexion and inversion of the foot • The patient will have pain in the medial lower leg • History and physical exam will correlate	• No diagnostic evidence available

Lateral Lower Leg Pain

Lateral Compartment Syndrome

HISTORY	MECHANISM OF INJURY	EVALUATION ESSENTIALS
• Patient reports tightness in lower leg and deep aching pain • Chronic or acute onset • Pain identified with activity that subsides when activity stops	• Acute occurs due a direct trauma • Chronic usually occurs with running and jumping activities at a certain point and in time during the activity • Acute exertional is typically not due to trauma; it can involve minimal to moderate trauma	• Assess tenderness to palpation • Inspect lower leg for distal pulse • Referral for pressure measurement • Evaluate muscle strength

KEY FINDINGS	DIAGNOSTIC EVIDENCE
• History will correlate to the physical exam • Pain is typically posterolateral • The patient will have pain, swelling, and neurological symptoms due to the structures in the lateral compartment	• Acute compartment intra-compartmental pressure monitoring (sensitivity 94%, specificity 98%)[16] • MRI for chronic compartment syndrome (sensitivity 96%, specificity 87%)[17]

Lateral Lower Leg Pain

Peroneal Neuropathy

HISTORY	MECHANISM OF INJURY	EVALUATION ESSENTIALS
• Patient reports an inability to lift ankle, extend toes, or turn foot out	• Traumatic associated with musculoskeletal injury or with isolated nerve traction, compression, or laceration • May occur as result of metabolic syndrome or mass lesion • Acute onset • Often from direct blow	• Assess AROM and PROM • Inspect gait • Evaluate muscle strength of the peroneal muscles including plantar flexion with eversion and dorsiflexion with eversion, as well as extensor muscles

KEY FINDINGS	DIAGNOSTIC EVIDENCE
• Patient will demonstrate drop foot during gait analysis • The patient will be unable to dorsiflex ankle, extend toes, or evert ankle	• MRI (accuracy ranging from 68% to 79%) and electrodiagnostic testing may be used to assist in evaluation[24]

Lateral Lower Leg Pain

Peroneal Strain

HISTORY	MECHANISM OF INJURY	EVALUATION ESSENTIALS
• Patient reports pain in the lateral lower leg • Acute onset • Pain identified with specific activity and then with ADLs	• Forceful eccentric contraction • Quick lateral move-ment	• Assess MMT for plantar flexion and eversion of the foot, as well as dorsiflexion and eversion • Inspect muscle and tendon

KEY FINDINGS	DIAGNOSTIC EVIDENCE
• The patient will have pain with plantar flexion or dorsiflexion with eversion of the foot • The patient will have pain in the lower leg and possibly swelling • History and physical exam will correlate	• No diagnostic evidence available.

Paper Patient—Lower Leg: Revisited

You should have been able to rule out several conditions secondary to knowing what structures are in the posterior lower leg. Your differential should have been Achilles tendinopathy versus gastrocnemius strain

Learning Activities: Practice Case

Use the blank templates provided in the appendices to write out a differential diagnosis map and clinical findings overview for the case provided below. When working with paper patients it is tempting to try to jump to "the answer" and come to a diagnosis. However the visual learning approach to differential diagnosis is designed to help you consider all the possibilities for the information provided. Good luck.

Paper Patient: Shin Pain in a New Runner

History

Andrea is a 20-year-old runner who reports that she is having medial shin pain from running. She started having pain during the start of the school year (2 months ago). She started a more robust running program during her semester break in order to lose some weight. She states that while she has always been a regular exerciser in the gym, she only recently started running. Andrea states that she runs 3 times a week and usually runs about 3 miles at a time. She has not run in the last week, and had to discontinue her last run due to pain. She feels better with rest, but pain always returns when she resumes running. She reports that she has good supportive running shoes that are only 1 month old. She describes a broad area of discomfort and denies pinpoint tenderness. She has pain with ADLs (walking) and reports a normal menstrual and nutritional profile.

Physical Exam

The physical exam reveals that Andrea has normal knee and ankle exams. She was tender over an area of medial tibia just superior to medial malleolus. MMT was 5/5 for all planes at the ankle and she reported pain (3/10) with resisted inversion and eversion. There was no pinpoint bony tenderness. Observation revealed a neutral foot alignment with normal arch height. Her core strength is poor because she cannot maintain a level position during a 20-second bridge challenge. MMT of the hip revealed 4/5 hip extension strength with all other planes 5/5 strength. PROM revealed tight posterior lower leg musculature with PROM dorsiflexion. Decreased joint play with a/p translation of the talus is noted. Her neurovascular exam is normal.

References

1. American Academy of Orthopaedic Surgeons. *The foot and ankle.* Available at http://orthoinfo.aaos.org/topic.cfm?topic=A00150. Retrieved on September 7, 2013.
2. McGuine TA, Keene JS. The effect of a balance training program on risk of ankle injury in high school athletes. *Am J Sports Med.* 2006;34:1103-1111.
3. US Consumers Product Safety Commission, Directorate of Economic Analysis. (2003).
4. Liu SH, Nuccion SL, Finerman G. Diagnosis of anterolateral ankle impingement. Comparison between magnetic resonance imaging and clinical examination. *Am J Sports Med.* 1997;25(3): 389-393.
5. Vaseenon T, Gao Y, Phisitkul P. Comparison of two manual tests for ankle laxity due to rupture of the lateral ankle ligaments. *Iowa Orthop J.* 2012;32:9-16.
6. de César PC, Avila EM, de Abreu MR. Comparison of magnetic resonance imaging to physical examination for syndesmotic injury after lateral ankle sprain. *Foot Ankle Int.* 2011;32(12):1110-1114.
7. Peduto AJ, Read JW. Imaging of ankle tendinopathy and tears. *Top Magn Reson Imaging.* 2010;21(1):25-36.
8. Bottger BA, Schweitzer ME, El-Noueam KI, Desai M. MR imaging of the normal and abnormal retrocalcaneal bursae. *AJR Am J Roentgenol.* 1998;170(5): 1239-1241.
9. Giannini S, Buda R, Mosca M, Parma A, Di Caprio F. Posterior ankle impingement. *Foot Ankle Int.* 2013;34(3):459-465.
10. Lynch SA. Assessment of the injured ankle in the athlete. *J Athl Train.* 2002;37(4):406-412.
11. Ahmad M, Tsang K, Mackenney PJ, Adedapo AO. Tarsal tunnel syndrome: A literature review. *Foot Ankle Surg.* 2012;18(3):149-152.
12. Premkumar A, Perry MB, Dwyer AJ, et al. Sonography and MR imaging of posterior tibial tendinopathy. *AJR Am J Roentgenol.* 2002;178(1):223-232.
13. Park HJ, Cha SD, Kim HS, et al. Reliability of MRI findings of peroneal tendinopathy in patients with lateral chronic ankle instability. *Clin Orthop Surg.* 2010;2(4):237-243.
14. Lee SJ, Jacobson JA, Kim SM, et al. Ultrasound and MRI of the peroneal tendons and associated pathology. *Skeletal Radiol.* 2013;42(9):1191-1200.
15. Roth JA, Taylor WC, Whalen J. Peroneal tendon subluxation: The other lateral ankle injury. *Br J Sports Med.* 2010;44(14):1047-1053.
16. McQueen MM, Duckworth AD, Aitken SA, Court-Brown CM. The estimated sensitivity and specificity of compartment pressure monitoring for acute compartment syndrome. *J Bone Joint Surg Am.* 2013;17;95(8):673-677.
17. Ringler MD, Litwiller DV, Felmlee JP, et al. MRI accurately detects chronic exertional compartment syndrome: A validation study. *Skeletal Radiol.* 2013;42(3):385-392.
18. Khan KM, Forster BB, Robinson J, et al. Are ultrasound and magnetic resonance imaging of value in assessment of Achilles tendon disorders? A two year prospective study. *Br J Sports Med.* 2003;37(2):149-154.
19. Asplund CA, Best TM. Achilles tendon disorders. *BMJ.* 2013;12:346.

20. Huisman MV, Klok FA. Diagnostic management of acute deep vein thrombosis and pulmonary embolism. *J Thromb Haemost.* 2013;11(3):412-422.
21. Hayashi D, Hamilton B, Guermazi A, de Villiers R, Crema MD, Roemer FW. Traumatic injuries of thigh and calf muscles in athletes: Role and clinical relevance of MR imaging and ultrasound. *Insights Imaging.* 2012;3(6):591-601.
22. Mansfield CJ, Beaumont J, Tarnay L, Silvers H. Popliteus strain with concurrent deltoid ligament sprain in an elite soccer athlete: A case report. *Int J Sports Phys Ther.* 2013;8(4):452-461.
23. Moen MH. Medial tibial stress syndrome: A critical review. *Sports Med.* 2009;39(7):523-546.
24. Lee PP, Chalian M, Bizzell C, et al. Magnetic resonance neurography of common peroneal (fibular) neuropathy. *J Comput Assist Tomogr.* 2012;36(4):455-461.

4

The Knee and Patellofemoral Joint

Injuries to the knee are becoming a pressing public health concern due to the economic costs associated with knee injury, the potential detrimental effects on health and wellness, and the risk of long-term osteoarthritis.[1,2] Injuries to the knee and patellofemoral joint are commonplace in sport and physical activity. In a study of high school athletes in the United States, Ingram et al[3] reported that, in adolescents, the knee joint is considered to be the second most commonly injured joint, accounting for 15.2% of all injuries; only the ankle accounted for more injuries (20.9%). The knee was the most common joint requiring surgery in that particular study (44.6%). Overall, it is estimated that knee surgeries alone account for nearly 60% of all sports-related surgeries.[3] Females who participate in structured sport or physical activities have been shown to have an incidence of knee injuries that is 3 to 6 times higher than their male counterparts.[4,5] In addition, recent literature indicates that the negative patient outcomes from knee injury are not isolated to those requiring surgery. When considering running injuries, the knee and patellofemoral joint are the most common location of injury; 20% of all running injuries occur at the knee, with iliotibial band syndrome and patellofemoral syndrome being the most common of these injuries.[6,7] Anterior knee pain injuries are more prevalent in female patients[8] and are associated with poor physical activity outcomes at 1-year follow up.[9]

Given the frequency of knee injuries in the sport and physical activity setting, coupled with the potential for negative long-term outcomes, the

Winterstein AP, Clark SV. *The Athletic Trainer's Guide to Differential Diagnosis (pp 87-122).*

ability of the athletic trainer to understand the wide range of possible diagnoses for the knee is essential for proper assessment, treatment, and referral. The diagnostic maps for the knee joint address issues of the tibiofemoral joint and the patellofemoral joint. The regional approach provides a clear and logical template for the clinician.

Paper Patient: Knee Pain in a Cyclist

History

Joe is a 54-year-old cyclist who comes to your clinic with a chief concern of posterolateral left knee pain and catching. He reports that he has always been tight in his muscles. He doesn't want to have surgery, so he is willing to do any exercises to get better quickly because cycling season is starting.

Physical Exam

On physical exam, you find that the patient is tender over the posteromedial joint line on the left. He also has tenderness over the semitendinosus on the left. Manual muscle testing (MMT) of the medial hamstrings reproduces pain. The patient has left knee pain with active motion from deep flexion to extension. Gluteus maximus and medius strength was 5/5 bilaterally. Hip external rotator strength on the left was 4/5 as compared to the right. Negative ligamentous testing. The patient had a positive Ober's and Thomas test. His standing alignment revealed mild navicular drop, mild calcaneal eversion, and genu varum.

Clinical Decisions

Using the information from your clinical exam, ask yourself these questions to guide your clinical decision making:

- What is your differential diagnosis?
- What key findings do you see to help guide your differential?
- What are the possible injuries associated with posterior and medial knee pain?

Start with a review of the anatomy maps and a thorough consideration of the possible injuries and conditions that are common to the knee. Use the differential diagnosis maps to guide your thought process and organize the possibilities. The organized synthesis of this information is the essence of clinical decision making. With practice, you will be able to draw your own differential diagnosis maps.

Anatomy Map: Knee

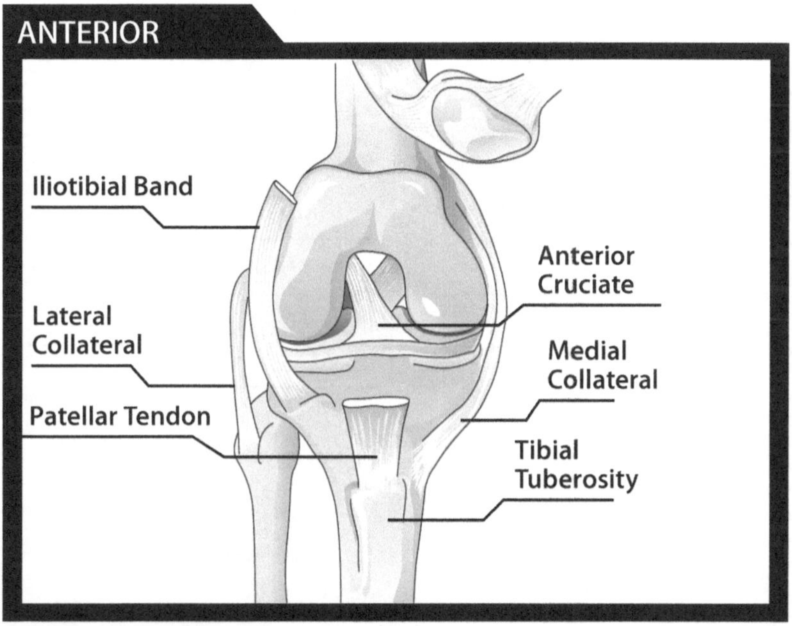

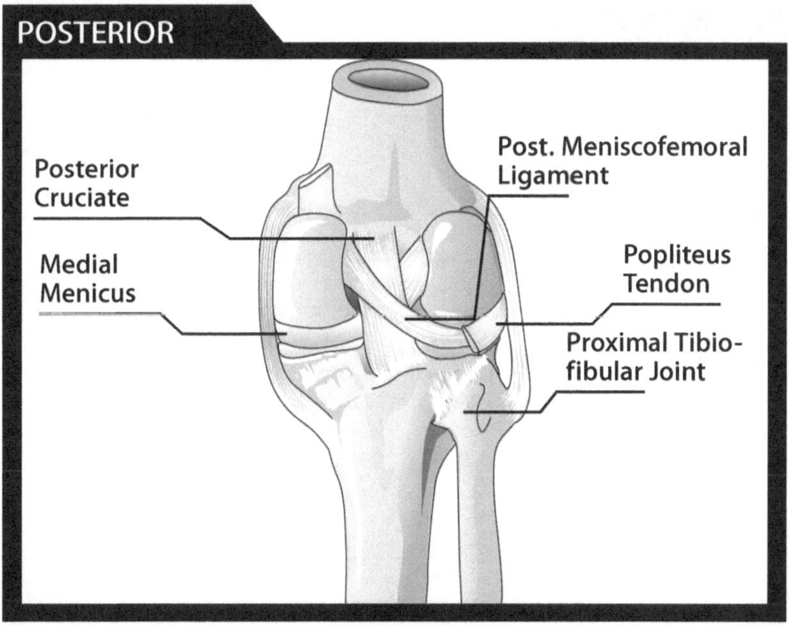

Anatomy Map: Knee

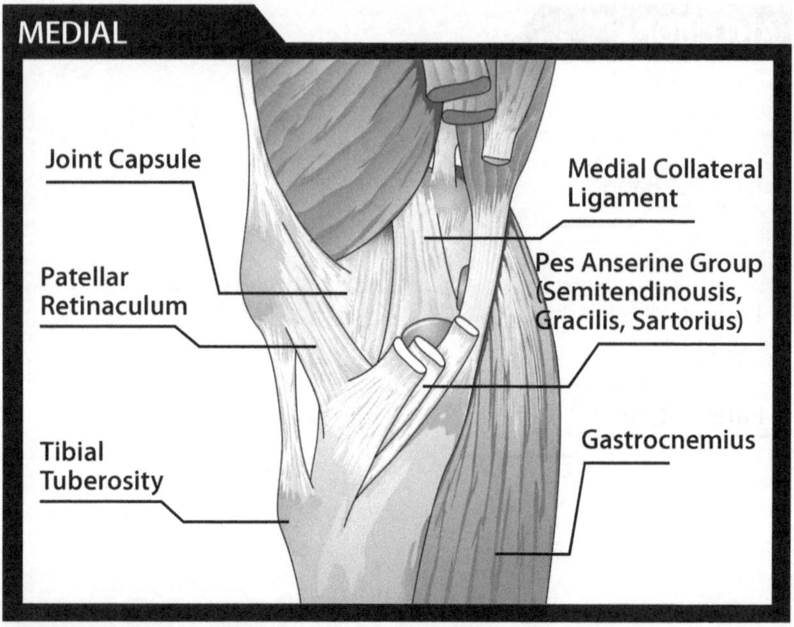

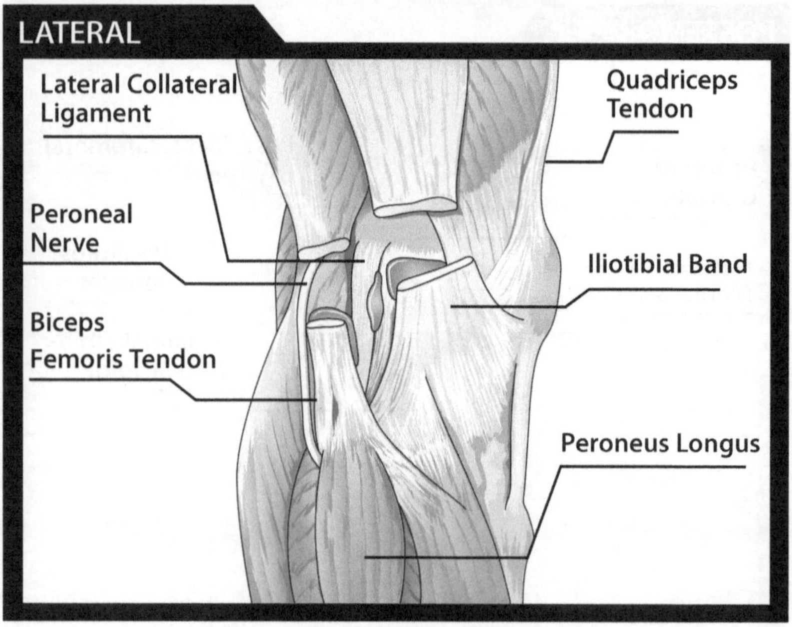

Knee Pain Map: Region/Soft Tissue Differential Diagnosis

ANTERIOR

- Anterior Cruciate Ligament (ACL) Sprain
- Fat Pad Impingement
- Osgood Schlatter's/ Tibial Apophysitis
- Patellar/Quadriceps Tendon Rupture
- Patellar/Quadriceps Tendonapothy
- Patellofemoral Syndrome (PFSS)
- Pes Anserine Bursitis
- Prepatellar Bursitis
- Sinding-Larson-Johannson Apophysitis

POSTERIOR

- Gastrocnemius Strain
- Proximal Hamstring Strain*
- Posterior Cruciate Ligament (PCL) Sprain
- Popliteal Cyst
- Posterior Horn Meniscal Tear
- Soleus Strain

Refer to Thigh Map (page 145)

MEDIAL

- Medial Collateral Ligament (MCL) Sprain
- Medial Meniscus Tear
- Medial Patellar Retinaculum Irritation
- Plica
- Semimembranosus/ Semitendinosus Tendinopathy
- Semimembranosus Strain
- Semitendiosus Strain

LATERAL

- Biceps Femoris Tendinopathy
- Biceps Femoris Strain
- Iliotibial Band (ITB) Friction Syndrome
- Lateral Meniscus Tear
- Lateral Collateral Ligament (LCL) Sprain
- Proximal Tibiofibular (Syndesmosis) Sprain

Knee Pain

Injuries to Bone/Joint Surfaces

COMMON FRACTURES

- Tibial plateau
- Tibial tuberosity avulsion (patellar tendon)
- Lateral tibial condyle avulsion (Segond)
- Femoral condyles
- Stieda fracture (avulsion of MC from femur)
- Pellegrini-Stieda (PS) lesion (ossification in or near the medial collateral ligament at medial femoral condyle)
- Distal shaft of femur
- Osteochondral lesion
- Osteochondritis dissecans
    - Arthroscopic Classification (Guhl)
    - Type I = softening of cartilage but no breach
    - Type II = breached cartilage that is stable
    - Type III = definable fragment that remains partially attached (flap lesion)
    - Type IV = loose body and osteochondral defect at the donor site
- Patella (bipartite patella is a common normal variant)
- Fibular head
- Proximal fibula (Maisonneuve)

Clinical Assessment of Knee Injuries

Anterior Knee Pain

Anterior Cruciate Ligament Sprain

HISTORY	MECHANISM OF INJURY	EVALUATION ESSENTIALS
• Patient may report a contact or noncontact injury mechanism • Patient may report a feeling of instability • A feeling of instability will be with 2 and 3; possibly pain • Patient may report an audible "pop" • A history of effusion (small or large) is common	• Planting and cutting with valgus load • Hyperextension • Deceleration plant with rotation • Injury may occur with contact or noncontact	• Lachman's test • Anterior drawer • Sweep test for effusion

KEY FINDINGS	DIAGNOSTIC EVIDENCE
• Audible pop • Presence of effusion • Sense of instability • Can occur with multiple ligament injuries (eg, MCL); comprehensive knee exam is essential • Grades 1 to 3 with 3 being full rupture • Symptoms vary depending upon the level of sprain	• Lachman's test (sensitivity 85%, specificity 94%) • Anterior drawer test (acute) (sensitivity 49%, specificity 52%) • Anterior drawer test (chronic) (sensitivity 92%, specificity 91%) • Pivot shift test (sensitivity 98%, specificity 24%)[10]

Anterior Knee Pain

Fat Pad Impingement

HISTORY	MECHANISM OF INJURY	EVALUATION ESSENTIALS
• Patient c/o pain with standing or hyperextension • Direct blow to anterior and inferior knee • Post surgical (ACL or arthoscopy) • Worse with jumping, running, or swimming	• Hyperextension injury • Direct blow • Post surgical	• ROM (hyperextension) of the knee • Overpressure to the inferior pole of the patella and quadriceps contraction • Movement analysis (squat) • MMT of quadriceps • Direct palpation

KEY FINDINGS	DIAGNOSTIC EVIDENCE
• TTP over the inferior pole of the patella across the tendon and beyond the borders either or both medially or laterally • Sometimes swelling of anterior/inferior knee around the fat pad	• MRI is the most accurate test to detect fat pad pathology[11]

Anterior Knee Pain

Osgood Schlatter's/Tibial Apophysitis

HISTORY	MECHANISM OF INJURY	EVALUATION ESSENTIALS
• Knee pain • Insidious onset • May present unilateral or bilateral • Patient may report recent growth spurt • Increased training volume or instensity • Pain with kneeling activities	• Repetitive running or jumping activities in growing adolescent	• Passive quadriceps stretching (knee flexion) • MMT for quadriceps • Palpation of tibial tubercle

KEY FINDINGS	DIAGNOSTIC EVIDENCE
• Increased bony growth at tubercle on palpation • Palpation is painful • Often visible bony growth • Weakness or pain with MMT • Radiographs may be ordered to determine if bony ossicle has separated from the tibia	• No diagnostic evidence available

Anterior Knee Pain

Patellar/Quadriceps Tendon Rupture

HISTORY	MECHANISM OF INJURY	EVALUATION ESSENTIALS
• History of chronic tendinopathy • Pain • Report of popping/ripping of the tendon • Swelling • Possible visible defect • Possible history of steriod abuse	• Eccentric loading • Deceleration	• MMT for knee extension • Direct palpation of tendon structures • Inspect for visible deformities

KEY FINDINGS	DIAGNOSTIC EVIDENCE
• Audible pop during injury • Visible bulk from retraction of muscle tissue • Palpable defect in tendon • MMT for knee extension reveals weakness and pain • Clinician must refrain from aggressive physical exam to prevent additional tissue damage • Clinical exam confirms suspected tendon rupture	• MRI is the most accurate diagnostic test • Radiograph is able to detect some ruptures by displacement of patella • Ultrasound is unreliable[11]

Anterior Knee Pain

Patellar/Quadriceps Tendinopathy

HISTORY	MECHANISM OF INJURY	EVALUATION ESSENTIALS
• Anterior knee pain • Pain may be present at inferior pole of patella, tibial tubercle, or superior patellar pole • Pain during activity better at rest than progressing to pain with ADLs • May have mild swelling	• Athletes who participate in repetitive jumping and kicking activities • Overloading of the extensor mechanism • Recent rapid increase in training volume and/or intensity	• Direct palpation • MMT • Passive knee flexion/quadriceps stretch • Thomas test

KEY FINDINGS	DIAGNOSTIC EVIDENCE
• Pain is focal • Loss of tissue mobility in quadriceps • Crepitus with MMT of the quadriceps in certain cases • Pain may progress to pain with ADLs and exacerbated by ascending stairs • Patients may report sensation of giving way; particularly in patients with quadriceps weakness	• MRI is the most accurate diagnostic test • Radiograph is able to detect some ruptures by displacement of patella • Ultrasound is unreliable[11]

Anterior Knee Pain

Patellofemoral Stress Syndrome

HISTORY	MECHANISM OF INJURY	EVALUATION ESSENTIALS
• General pain about the patella and posterior to patella with squatting or sitting for long periods of time • Pain with running activities	• Recent increases in volume and/or intensity of activities • May occur after recent growth spurt • Post operative onset when quadriceps and other muscles are tight and weak	• Patellar mobility testing • MMT for muscles surrounding knee • Positive Thomas for hip flexors • Ober's test for ITB • Hamstring flexibility tests • Gait analysis

KEY FINDINGS	DIAGNOSTIC EVIDENCE
• Common to growing adolescents; can continue into adulthood • Little to no swelling • Hypermobile patella • Tight lateral patellar structures are common finding (positive Ober's test) • Loss of soft tissue mobility • Patellofermoral issues are multifactorial and require a comprehensive evaluation	• Pain with squat (sensitivity 95%, specificity 50%) • Vastus medialis coordination test (sensitivity 16%, specificity 93%) • Clarke's test (sensitivity 48%, specificity 75%) • Patellar tilt (sensitivity 43%, specificity 92%) • Medial patellar tenderness (sensitivity 48%, specificity 71%)[13]

Anterior Knee Pain

Pes Anserine Bursitits

HISTORY

- Anterior/medial knee pain
- Pain going up and down the stairs
- Local swelling of the bursa
- Pain changing positions from sitting to standing

MECHANISM OF INJURY

- Repetitive activity
- Recent rapid increase in training volume and/or intensity

EVALUATION ESSENTIALS

- MMT gracilis, semitendinosus, and sartorius
- Loss of tissue mobility in muscles of the pes group
- Direct palpation of over pes group tendons
- Visible inspection for swelling of bursa

KEY FINDINGS

- Tender to direct palpation
- Common in distance runners
- Common in females (more adult cases compared to younger populations)
- Common with osteoarthritis, rheumatoid arthritis, obese, and diabetic patients
- Comprehensive evaluation should also examine ankle motion and overall LE biomechanics

DIAGNOSTIC EVIDENCE

- No diagnostic evidence available

Anterior Knee Pain

Prepatellar Bursitis

HISTORY	MECHANISM OF INJURY	EVALUATION ESSENTIALS
• Patient reports an acute injury such as a fall or collision • Chronic onset from repetitive kneeling • Pain	• Direct blow to prepatellar region • Repetitive kneeling	• Ballotable patella • Inspect for swelling of the bursa • Palpation • Assess ROM • MMT

KEY FINDINGS	DIAGNOSTIC EVIDENCE
• Erythema with immediate extracellular swelling • Tender to palpation • Loss of motion/pain with motion • Muscular inhibition secondary to swelling • Bursa must be watched closely for infection • Recurrence is common; padding can aid in preventing recurrent injury	• No diagnostic evidence available

Anterior Knee Pain

Sinding-Larsen-Johansson (Apophysitis)

HISTORY	MECHANISM OF INJURY	EVALUATION ESSENTIALS
• Patient c/o pain and swelling at distial pole of the patella and patellar tendon • Insidious onset • Recent growth spurt • Increased training volume and intensity • Pain with ascending stairs • Pain with stretching quads	• Overuse and repetitive stress • Recent growth spurt • Training errors • Recent rapid increase in training volume and/or intensity	• Direct palpation to inferior pole of the patella • ROM (passive knee flexion and stretching of the quads) • MMT

KEY FINDINGS	DIAGNOSTIC EVIDENCE
• Palpation is painful at inferior pole of the patella • Passive stretching of the knee in flexion reproduced pain • Pain with MMT or activation of quads • Radiographs may be ordered to determine if bony ossicle has separated from the pole ot the patella	• No diagnostic evidence available

Posterior Knee Pain

Gastrocnemius Strain

HISTORY	MECHANISM OF INJURY	EVALUATION ESSENTIALS
• Patient describes pain in the calf • Pain with push off • Posterior knee pain • A sensation of tightness and stiffness • Patient reports swelling	• Knee extension with dorsiflexion of the ankle	• Palpation of the medial and lateral gastroc heads • MMT of the gastrocnemius with straight leg

KEY FINDINGS	DIAGNOSTIC EVIDENCE
• The gastrocnemius strain is more typical than a soleus strain • Important to evaluate with knee in extension versus flexion to differentiate gastrocnemius from soleus • Symptoms vary depending on severity of the strain	• MRI can be useful to evaluate extent of muscle damage • New evidence shows that MRI may be able to help predict time required to return to athletic competition • Ultrasound less accurate than MRI for diagnostic assessment[14]

Posterior Knee Pain

Posterior Cruciate Ligament Sprain

HISTORY

- Patients may report a feeling of subtle instability with third degree sprain
- Patient describes a mechanism consistent with PCL injury
- Possible effusion
- May hear "pop"

MECHANISM OF INJURY

- Fall on flexed knee
- Flexed knee impact
- Forced hyperflexion of the knee with foot plantarflexed
- Less commonly hyperextension

EVALUATION ESSENTIALS

- Posterior tibial sag (Godfrey's test)
- Posterior drawer
- Reverse pivot shift
- Step off deformity at the tibia

KEY FINDINGS

- Clinical exam findings consistent with patient history
- Patient may hear "pop" but don't feel the instability so they often want to return to play
- Mild to moderate effusion 2 to 6 hours post-injury
- Fun fact: the PCL is the strongest ligament in the knee
- Grades 1 to 3 with 3 being full rupture
- Symptoms vary depending upon the level of sprain

DIAGNOSTIC EVIDENCE

- Posterior sag (sensitivity 79%, specificity 100%)
- Posterior drawer (sensitivity 51% to 90%, specificity 99%)
- Quadriceps activation test (sensitivity 54% to 98%, specificity 97% to 100%)[15]

Posterior Knee Pain

Popliteal Cyst

HISTORY	MECHANISM OF INJURY	EVALUATION ESSENTIALS
• Patient may or may not describe pain in the posterior knee • Patient describes a fullness in the posterior knee • Knee motion may be limited	• Non-specific mechanism • Cysts often form secondary to swelling • Maybe associated with swelling secondary to arthritis	• Palpation of soft mass in popliteal space (posterior knee)

KEY FINDINGS	DIAGNOSTIC EVIDENCE
• Popliteal cysts are also called a Baker's cyst (named after William Morrant Baker [1839 to 1896]) who described the condition • Symptoms can mimic meniscal tears	• MRI is useful to correctly identify the type of cyst and other potential contributing factors • Baker's cyst has incidence of 38%[16]

Posterior Knee Pain

Posterior Horn Meniscal Tear

HISTORY	MECHANISM OF INJURY	EVALUATION ESSENTIALS
• Patient reports posteromedial or posterolateral knee pain • Description of clicking, catching, or giving way type symptoms • May describe effusion • Pain with deep flexion	• Planted foot with rotation • Deep flexion with rotation • Acute MOI or insidious symptoms from chronic meniscal degeneration	• McMurray's or Thessaly test for meniscus • Assessment of deep knee flexion • Palpation of pain along the joint line • Sweep test for possible effusion

KEY FINDINGS	DIAGNOSTIC EVIDENCE
• These types of meniscal tears are typically seen in the aging population with or without a specific mechanism	• Joint line tenderness (sensitivity 64%, specificity 61%) • McMurray's test (sensitivity 51%, specificity 78%) • Thessaly test (sensitivity 91%, specificity 94%)[17]

Posterior Knee Pain

Soleus Strain

HISTORY	MECHANISM OF INJURY	EVALUATION ESSENTIALS
• Patient describes calf pain (lateral) • Reports of calf tightness • Pain worsens over time • Walking or jogging brings on symptoms	• Knee flexed with dorsiflexion of the ankle	• Palpation of the medial and lateral gastroc • MMT of the soleus with knee flexed

KEY FINDINGS	DIAGNOSTIC EVIDENCE
• The soleus strain is less typical than the gastrocnemius strain • Clinicians must remember to palpate the lateral side all along gastrocnemius and MMT with flexed knee • Swelling not typical • Symptoms vary depending upon the grade of sprain	• MRI can be useful to evaluate extent of muscle damage • New evidence shows that MRI may be able to help predict time required to return to athletic competition • Ultrasound less accurate than MRI for diagnostic assessment[14]

Medial Knee Pain

Medial Collateral Sprain

HISTORY	MECHANISM OF INJURY	EVALUATION ESSENTIALS
• Acute trauma • Medial knee pain along the path of the MCL • Patient reports injury with fixed foot position and a direct blow to the lateral aspect of the knee	• Valgus force to the knee • Foot fixed and direct blow • Can be injured by external tibial rotation (rare)	• Straight plane ligament test with a valgus force • MCL is isolated in partial flexion (25 to 30 degrees) • Laxity in full extension may indicate capsular or cruciate involvement • Direct palpation

KEY FINDINGS	DIAGNOSTIC EVIDENCE
• Painful gait • Pain in side to side movements that recreate valgus force • Pain with direct palpation • Loss of motion (terminal extension and terminal flexion) secondary to pain • Other knee structures must be ruled out (medial meniscus and cruciates)	• No conclusive supporting evidence is reported for valgus testing of the knee • Clinically, valgus testing is considered to be helpful for identifying this clinical condition

Medial Knee Pain

Medial Meniscus Tear

HISTORY	MECHANISM OF INJURY	EVALUATION ESSENTIALS
• May present as acute injury or gradual onset • Patient reports medial joint line pain • Patient may report effusion • Patient may report sensations of instability, clicking, or catching/locking in the knee joint	• Accumulated trauma in gradual onset injuries • Tibial rotation in combination with flexion and extension; may include varus or valgus loads • Hyperflexion and hyperextension of the knee can impinge the anterior and posterior horns of the meniscus	• Palpation of the joint line • McMurray's and Thessaly test for meniscus • ROM assessment

KEY FINDINGS	DIAGNOSTIC EVIDENCE
• Mechanical symptoms consistent with physical exam findings • Presence of effusion • While isolated meniscal tears are common, all other ligamentous and capsular injuries must be ruled out as the medial meniscus has an anatomical attachment to the MCL/joint capsule	• McMurray's test (sensitivity 51%, specificity 78%) • Joint line tenderness (sensitivity 64%, specificity 61%) • Thessaly test (sensitivity 91%, specificity 97%) • The Thessaly test is most sensitive and specific in the absence of other knee pathology[17]

Medial Knee Pain

Medial Patellar Retinaculum Irritation

HISTORY	MECHANISM OF INJURY	EVALUATION ESSENTIALS
• Gradual onset • Rapid changes in intensity and volume of activity • Patient complains of anterior-medial knee pain • Pain with knee flexion and extension • Pain with long periods of sitting • Pain with use of stairs	• Gradual onset • Overuse • Repetitive activities • Recent rapid increase in training volume and/or intensity	• Assess Q angle • MMT for quads and hips (abduction, external rotation, and extension) • Patellar mobility assessment • Direct palpation

KEY FINDINGS	DIAGNOSTIC EVIDENCE
• Associated with PFSS and subluxing patella • Tension on medial structures as patella is pulled laterally • Evaluation of hip and core strength is essential for comprehensive assessment • Weakness in hip abduction, external rotation, and extension • Quad weakness	• High resolution MRI can be used to assess various layers of the retinaculum • Fibrosis, thickening, and ossification of the retinaculum can be identified via MRI[18]

Medial Knee Pain

Plica

HISTORY	MECHANISM OF INJURY	EVALUATION ESSENTIALS
• Patient reports mild to severe pain with activity • Acute or chronic onset • Pain identified with ascending or descending the stairs	• Repetitive flexion of the knee during activities causing impingement of the plica between the patella and medial femoral condyle • Direct trauma to the medial knee	• Mediopatellar plica (MPP) test • Palpation of the medial plica and possible effusion • Arthroscopy is the gold standard test

KEY FINDINGS	DIAGNOSTIC EVIDENCE
• The patient will have pain over the plica on palpation • Palpable snap or crepitus • Possible knee joint effusion • Medial plica syndrome is the most common of the plicae about the knee	• MPP test (sensitivity 90%, specificity 89%) • Ultrasound (sensitivity 90%, specificity 83%) • MRI (sensitivity 77%, specificity 58%)[19]

Medial Knee Pain

Semimembranosus/Semitendinosus Tendinopathy

HISTORY	MECHANISM OF INJURY	EVALUATION ESSENTIALS
• Gradual onset • Patient reports changes in training volume and/or intensity • Pain at medial and posterior-medial corner of the knee • Patient may report crepitus	• Repetitive deceleration activities with eccentric load • Repetitive flexion activities • Rapid increases in activities	• Palpation along the semimembranosus or semitendinosus tendons at insertion • MMT • ROM

KEY FINDINGS	DIAGNOSTIC EVIDENCE
• Crepitus along the distal tendons • Semitendinosus pain may refer to the conjoined tendons of the pes anserine • Passive knee extension may cause pain	• Research reveals mixed results in the efficacy of ultrasound and MRI in diagnostic evaluation for tendinopathy[20]

Medial Knee Pain

Semimembranosus Strain

HISTORY	MECHANISM OF INJURY	EVALUATION ESSENTIALS
• Sprinting, jumping, and landing activities • Patient reports pain in muscle or musculotendinous junction • Acute onset with possible popping sensation	• Rapid acceleration or deceleration movements • Eccentric loading on muscle tissue	• MMT in knee flexion • ROM • Palpation along the semimembranosus muscle and muscle-tendon junction

KEY FINDINGS	DIAGNOSTIC EVIDENCE
• Painful gait • Pain may refer to the posterior-medial aspect of the knee • Possible palpable defect in muscle tissue • Pain with active knee flexion and active hip extension with knee in extension • Pain with passive hip flexion and passive knee extension	• MRI can be used for severe injuries (sensitivity 33% to 100%, specificity 92% to 100%) • Diagnostic ultrasound for muscle strain evaluation (sensitivity 79% to 100%, specificity 92%)[20] • Predisposing factors include increased age, previous hamstring injury, fatigue, decreased flexibility, and muscle imbalance[21]

Medial Knee Pain

Semitendinosus Strain

HISTORY	MECHANISM OF INJURY	EVALUATION ESSENTIALS
• Sprinting, jumping, and landing activities • Patient reports pain in muscle or muscle-tendon junction • Acute onset with possible popping sensation	• Rapid acceleration or deceleration movements • Eccentric loading on muscle tissue	• MMT in knee flexion • Palpation along the semitendinosus muscle and muscle-tendon junction • ROM

KEY FINDINGS	DIAGNOSTIC EVIDENCE
• Painful gait • Pain may refer to the posterior-medial aspect of the knee • Possible palpable defect in muscle tissue • Pain with active knee flexion and active hip extension with knee in extension • Pain with passive hip flexion and passive knee extension	• MRI can be used for severe injuries (sensitivity 33% to 100%, specificity 92% to 100%) • Diagnostic ultrasound for muscle strain evaluation (sensitivity 79% to 100%, specificity 92%)[20] • Predisposing factors include increased age, previous hamstring injury, fatigue, decreased flexibility, and muscle imbalance[21]

Lateral Knee Pain

Biceps Femoris Tendinopathy

HISTORY	MECHANISM OF INJURY	EVALUATION ESSENTIALS
• Gradual onset • Patient reports changes in training volume and/or intensity • Pain at lateral and posterolateral aspect of the knee • Patient may report crepitus	• Repetitive deceleration activities with eccentric load • Repetitive flexion activities • Rapid increases in activities	• Palpation along the biceps femoris tendon at insertion • MMT • ROM at knee and hip

KEY FINDINGS	DIAGNOSTIC EVIDENCE
• Crepitus along the distal tendons • Passive knee extension may cause pain • Weakness with MMT secondary to pain	• Research reveals mixed results in the efficacy of ultrasound and MRI in diagnostic evaluation for tendinopathy[20]

Lateral Knee Pain

Biceps Femoris Strain

HISTORY	MECHANISM OF INJURY	EVALUATION ESSENTIALS
• Sprinting, jumping, and landing activities • Patient reports pain in muscle or muscle-tendon junction • Acute onset with possible popping sensation	• Rapid acceleration or deceleration movements • Eccentric load on muscle tissue	• MMT in knee flexion • Direct palpation to biceps femoris muscle and muscle-tendon where it inserts on the fibular head

KEY FINDINGS	DIAGNOSTIC EVIDENCE
• Painful gait • Pain may refer to the posterior-lateral aspect of the knee • Possible palpable defect in muscle tissue • Pain and/or weakness MMT of knee flexion and hip extension with knee in extension • Pain with passive hip flexion and passive knee extension	• MRI can be used for severe injuries (sensitivity 33% to 100%, specificity 92% to 100%) • Diagnostic ultrasound for muscle strain evaluation (sensitivity 79% to 100%, specificity 92%)[20] • Predisposing factors include: increased age, previous hamstring injury, fatigue, decreased flexibility, and muscle imbalance[21]

Lateral Knee Pain

Iliotibial Band Syndrome

HISTORY	MECHANISM OF INJURY	EVALUATION ESSENTIALS
• Gradual onset • Pain over the lateral epicondyle of femur at the distal portion of the ITB where it crosses the joint line • Rapid increase in running activities • Running the same direction or on the same side of the road	• Repetitive flexion and extension activities • Overuse	• Ober's test for ITB • Noble's compression test • Palpation of the distal ITB • ROM • Gait analysis

KEY FINDINGS	DIAGNOSTIC EVIDENCE
• Loss of mobility of ITB, over pronation, hip weakness, core weakness, and varum knee posture may contribute to this condition • Positive Ober's test and Noble's compression test • Tender to palpation	• Ober's test: limited evidence. Intratester reliability: 0.90 • Noble's compression test: absent in the literature. This test is anecdotally considered to be helpful for identifying pain in the ITB.[22]

Lateral Knee Pain

Lateral Meniscus Tear

HISTORY	MECHANISM OF INJURY	EVALUATION ESSENTIALS
• May present as acute injury or gradual onset • Patient reports lateral joint line pain • Patient may report effusion • Patient may report sensations of instability, clicking, or catching/locking in the knee joint	• Accumulated trauma in gradual onset injuries • Tibial rotation in combination with flexion and extension; may include varus/valgus loads • Hyperflexion and hyperextension of the knee can impinge the anterior and posterior horns of the meniscus	• Palpation of joint line • McMurray's and Thessaly test • ROM assessment

KEY FINDINGS	DIAGNOSTIC EVIDENCE
• Mechanical symptoms consistent with physical exam findings • Presence of effusion • Isolated meniscal tears are common, however, other ligamentous injury should be ruled out	• Joint line tenderness (sensitivity 64%, specificity 61%) • McMurray's test (sensitivity 51%, specificity 78%) • Thessaly test (sensitivity 91%, specificity 94%)[17]

Lateral Knee Pain

Lateral Collateral Sprain

HISTORY	MECHANISM OF INJURY	EVALUATION ESSENTIALS
• Acute trauma • Lateral knee pain along LCL from femoral condyle to fibular head • Varus force to the knee (eg, direct blow with foot fixed, landed on in pile up)	• Varus forces • Excess internal rotation of the tibia	• Straight plane ligament test with a varus force • LCL is isolated in partial flexion (25 to 30 degrees) • Laxity in full extension may indicate capsular or cruciate involvement • Direct palpation

KEY FINDINGS	DIAGNOSTIC EVIDENCE
• Other knee structures must be ruled out (meniscus and cruciate ligaments) • Bilateral comparison is essential given to assess normal variations in laxity • Adolescent patients must be carefully evaluated for epiphyseal involvement	• No conclusive supporting evidence is reported for valgus testing of the knee • Varus testing is generally considered to be helpful for identifying this clinical condition

Lateral Knee Pain

Proximal Tibiofibular (Syndesmosis) Sprain

HISTORY	MECHANISM OF INJURY	EVALUATION ESSENTIALS
• Pain over the fibular head and proximal fibula • Direct blow or inversion and plantar flexion ankle injury with associated knee flexion • Acute or insidious onset • Chronic may have bilateral discomfort and generalized laxity	• Associated ankle injury (inversion and plantar flexion) with knee flexed • Landing and twisting activities may increase risk of subluxation of dislocation	• Palpation at the proximal fibula • Stability assessment of proximal tib-fib joint (anterior/posterior) • Visible inspection • Gait analysis

KEY FINDINGS	DIAGNOSTIC EVIDENCE
• Pain with stability test and direct palpation • This joint is inherently stable. Injuries to this joint can sometimes be overlooked. • Ankle motions may exacerbate pain in the proximal fibula • Must rule out Maisonneuve fracture with lateral knee/fibula pain secondary to ankle MOI	• No diagnostic evidence available

Paper Patient: Revisited

Using the anatomy maps, differential diagnosis map, and a careful consideration of the possibilities, you should have been able to rule out several conditions secondary to knowing what structures are at the posterior knee. Your differential should have been lateral meniscal tear versus hamstring strain.

Learning Activities: Practice Case

Use the blank templates provided in the Appendices to write out a differential diagnosis map and clinical findings overview for the case provided below. When working with paper patients, it is tempting to try to jump to "the answer" and come to a diagnosis. However, the visual learning approach to differential diagnosis is designed to help you consider all the possibilities for the information provided. Good luck.

Paper Patient: Knee Pain in a College Student

History

Alfred is a 19-year-old college student who presents in clinic after falling out of his loft bed and hitting the ground. He also reports having some sleepwalking issues. Alfred is unsure of what happened. He had been at his fraternity that evening but denies drinking or having any impairment to his judgment. He points to the lateral joint line as his area of concern but describes a "deep pain." He states that his knee feels unstable in certain positions and he describes a sensation of giving way. He has no previous history of knee injury.

Physical Exam

The physical exam reveals a trace effusion. The patient is tender to palpation over the lateral condyle of the knee. Muscle guarding is preventing a quality examination of the ACL by Lachman's or anterior drawer. The step-off is normal and the posterior drawer test is negative. Varus and valgus stress tests are negative. He exhibits good muscle tone and muscle activation. AROM is WNL but painful (4/10) in knee flexion. There are visible abrasions on the patella and the surrounding tissue.

References

1. Louw QA, Manilall J, Grimmer KA. Epidemiology of knee injuries among adolescents: A systematic review. *Br J Sports Med.* 2008;42(1):2-10.
2. Button K, van Deursen R, Price P. Measurement of functional recovery in individuals with acute anterior cruciate ligament rupture. *Br J Sports Med.* 2005;39(11):866-71; discussion 866-71.
3. Ingram JG, Fields SK, Yard EE, Comstock RD. Epidemiology of knee injuries among boys and girls in US high school athletics. *Am J Sports Med.* 2008;36(6):1116-1122.
4. Arendt EA, Agel J, Dick R. Anterior cruciate ligament injury patterns among collegiate men and women. *J Athl Train.* 1999;34(2):86-92.
5. Dick R, Putukian M, Agel J, Evans TA, Marshall SW. Descriptive epidemiology of collegiate women's soccer injuries: National collegiate athletic association injury surveillance system, 1988-1989 through 2002-2003. *J Athl Train.* 2007;42(2):278-285.
6. Fields KB. Running injuries: Changing trends and demographics. *Curr Sports Med Rep.* 2011;10(5):299-303.
7. McKean KA, Manson NA, Stanish WD. Musculoskeletal injury in the masters runners. *Clin J Sports Med.* 2006; 16(12):149-154.
8. Boling M, Padua D, Marshall S, Guskiewicz K, Pyne S, Beutler A. Gender differences in the incidence and prevalence of patellofemoral pain syndrome. *Scand J Med Sci Sports.* 2010;20(5):725-730.
9. Winterstein AP, McGuine TM, Carr KE, Hetzel S. Changes in self-reported physical activity following knee injury in active females. *Athletic Training & Sports Health Care.* 2013;5(3):106-114.
10. Benjaminse A, Gokeler A, van der Schans CP. Clinical diagnosis of an anterior cruciate ligament rupture: A meta-analysis. *J Orthop Sports Phys Ther.* 2006;36(5):267-288.
11. Dragoo JL, Johnson C, McConnell J. Evaluation and treatment of disorders of the infrapatellar fat pad. *Sports Med.* 2012;42(1):51-67.
12. Swamy GN, Nanjayan SK, Yallappa S, Bishnoi A, Pickering SA. Is ultrasound diagnosis reliable in acute extensor tendon injuries of the knee? *Acta Orthop Belg.* 2012;78(6):764-770.
13. Nunes GS, Stapait EL, Kirsten MH, de Noronha M, Santos GM. Clinical test for diagnosis of patellofemoral pain syndrome: Systematic review with meta-analysis. *Phys Ther Sport.* 2013;14(1):54-59.
14. Hayashi D, Hamilton B, Guermazi A, de Villiers R, Crema MD, Roemer FW. Traumatic injuries of thigh and calf muscles in athletes: Role and clinical relevance of MR imaging and ultrasound. *Insights Imaging.* 2012;3(6):591-601.
15. Malanga GA, Andrus S, Nadler SF, McLean J. Physical examination of the knee: A review of the original test description and scientific validity of common orthopedic tests. *Arch Phys Med Rehabil.* 2003;84(4):592-603.
16. Perdikakis E, Skiadas V. MRI characteristics of cysts and "cyst-like" lesions in and around the knee: What the radiologist needs to know. *Insights Imaging.* 2013;4(3):257-272.
17. Ockert B, Haasters F, Polzer H, et al. Value of the clinical examination in suspected meniscal injuries. A meta-analysis. *Unfallchirurg.* 2010;113(4):293-299.
18. Thawait SK, Soldatos T, Thawait GK, Cosgarea AJ, Carrino JA, Chhabra A. High resolution magnetic resonance imaging of the patellar retinaculum: Normal anatomy, common injury patterns, and pathologies. *Skeletal Radiol.* 2012;41(2):137-148.

19. Stubbings N, Smith T. Diagnostic test accuracy of clinical and radiological assessments for medial patellar plica syndrome: A systematic review and meta-analysis. *Knee.* 2013 Nov 13. pii: S0968-0160(13)00211-1. doi: 10.1016/j.knee.2013.11.001. [Epub ahead of print].
20. Hodgson RJ, O'Connor PJ, Grainger AJ. Tendon and ligament imaging. *Br J Radiol.* 2012;85(1016):1157-1172.
21. Heiderscheit BC, Sherry MA, Silder A, Chumanov ES, Thelen DG. Hamstring strain injuries: Recommendations for diagnosis, rehabilitation, and injury prevention. *J Orthop Sports Phys Ther.* 2010;40(2):67-81.
22. Reese NB, Bandy WD. Use of an inclinometer to measure flexibility of the iliotibial band using the ober test and the modified ober test: Differences in magnitude and reliability of measurements. *J Orthop Sports Phys Ther.* 2003;33(6):326-330.

5

The Hip

Clinical assessment of the hip, femur, and pelvis presents the clinician with an array of evaluative challenges. This region contains large muscle groups that are frequently injured in sport and physical activity (eg, hamstrings, hip flexors, and quadriceps) and also is home to musculature that is associated with chronic injuries in the lower extremity (eg, weakness of the gluteal muscle group). To confound these challenges, the hip is a common location for referred pain from the pelvis and spine. In addition, clinicians must recognize that hip injuries can include serious joint injury, such as dislocations and fractures. Chronic hip joint pain can originate from the surrounding soft tissue (eg, snapping hip or proximal iliotibial [IT] band syndrome), from the joint itself (femoral acetabular impingement [FAI] or labral tears). While FAI and labral pathology have been documented for decades, improved clinical assessment and imaging techniques have helped identify these chronic joint injuries and led to an increase in their presentation clinically.[1]

When differentiating a potential diagnosis for injuries to the hip, it is important to understand injuries common to specific patient populations. Apophyseal injuries of the pelvis are most commonly due to sport participation and are frequently seen in adolescent boys. These injuries range from irritation of the apophysis (eg, apophysitis) to avulsion fractures of the secondary growth center. These bony avulsions occur at muscular origin and insertion points. The most common location of acute avulsion fracture

Winterstein AP, Clark SV. *The Athletic Trainer's Guide to Differential Diagnosis (pp 123-156).*

is the ischial tuberosity, followed by the anterior inferior iliac spine (AIIS), and anterior superior iliac spine (ASIS). Avulsions of the lesser trochanter are also fairly common, whereas iliac crest and pubic symphysis avulsions tend to be less frequent.[2] Differentiating these injuries from surrounding soft tissue injury is an essential part of a thorough assessment.

Injury rates for the hip and pelvis vary. Powell and Barber-Ross[3] presented injury rates for a group of boys and girls in interscholastic sports that range from 5.4% to 28.0% of all reported injuries. This variability is determined by sport type. When considering specific sports, injuries to the hip and thigh become more prominent. In an 11-year study of men's intercollegiate soccer injuries, Agel[4] reported 18% of all injuries in practice were to the hip/pelvis and thigh (8.2% muscle tendon strains to the thigh, 6.4% contusions to the thigh, and 3.9% muscle tendon injuries to the hip and pelvis). Injuries in games represented 24.4% of all reported injuries (16.6% to the thigh and 7.8% to the hip/pelvis).

Well-prepared clinicians dealing with active patients will need to be able to evaluate a range of thigh, hip, and pelvis injuries and conditions. The anatomy of the hip lends itself well to the regional body part approach and allows clinicians and students to use the visual approach to map potential injuries and attentively differentiate the diagnosis.

Paper Patient: Hip Pain in a Gymnast

History

Kate is a 13-year-old female gymnast and soccer player who presents with a chief complaint of anterior hip pain and popping of the left hip. It is specific to when she is doing her routine on the uneven bars.

Physical Exam

Her physical exam reveals no tenderness to palpation at the hip. Her MMT demonstrated 4/5 weakness over the gluteals, hamstrings, and hip external rotators. She has a history of a recent growth spurt. There is no pain with passive motion; however, active hip flexion to extension produces pain and snapping. The following tests are negative: FABER, FADIR, and hip scouring. The patient has pain and popping with passive deep hip flexion with rotation into external rotation.

Clinical Decisions

Using the information from your clinical exam, ask yourself these questions to guide your clinical decision making:

- What is your differential diagnosis?
- What key findings do you see to help guide your differential?
- What are the possible injuries associated with anterior hip pain?

Start with a review of the anatomy maps and a thorough consideration of the possible injuries and conditions that are common to the hip. Use the differential diagnosis maps to guide your thought process and organize the possibilities. The organized synthesis of this information is the essence of clinical decision making.

Anatomy Map: Hip

ANTERIOR

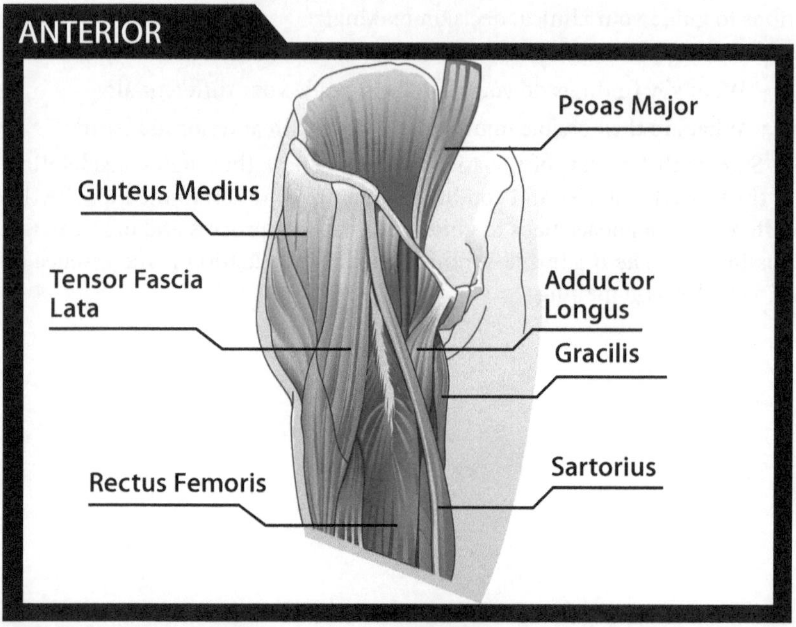

POSTERIOR

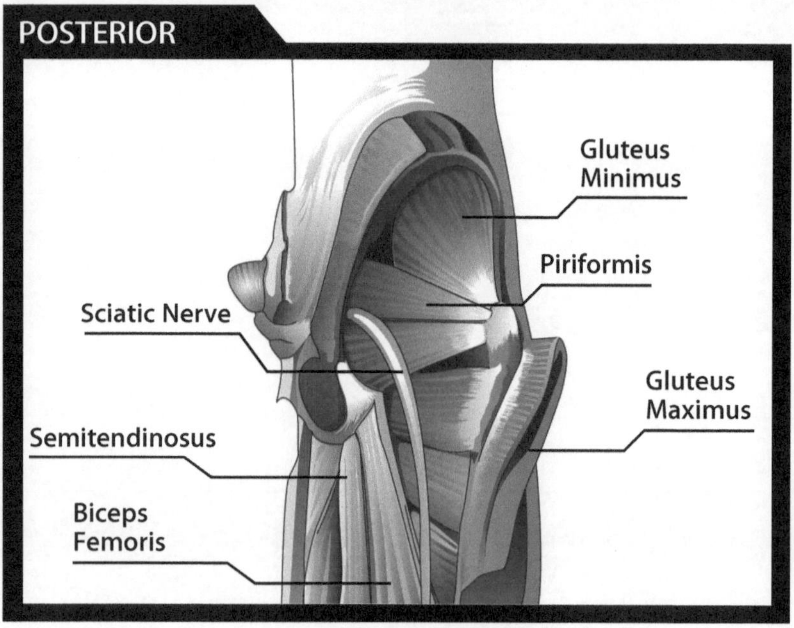

Anatomy Map: Hip

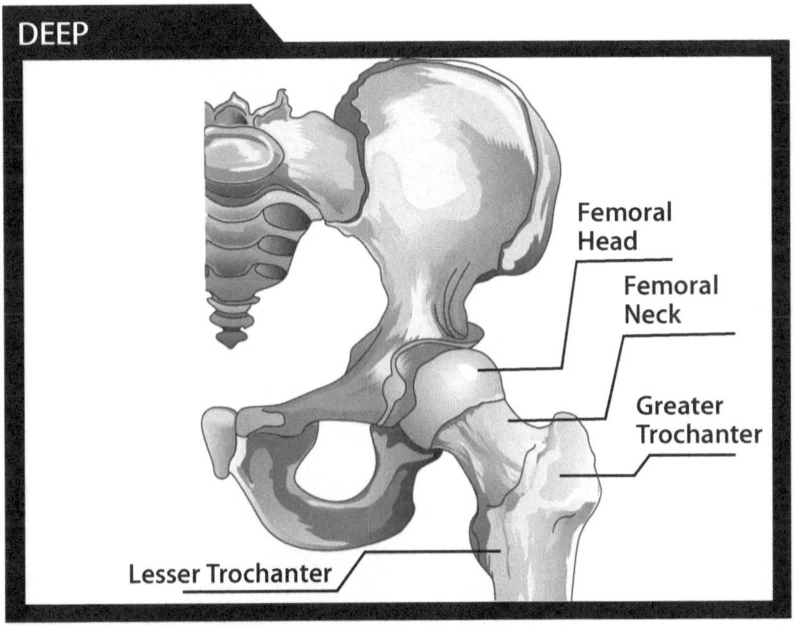

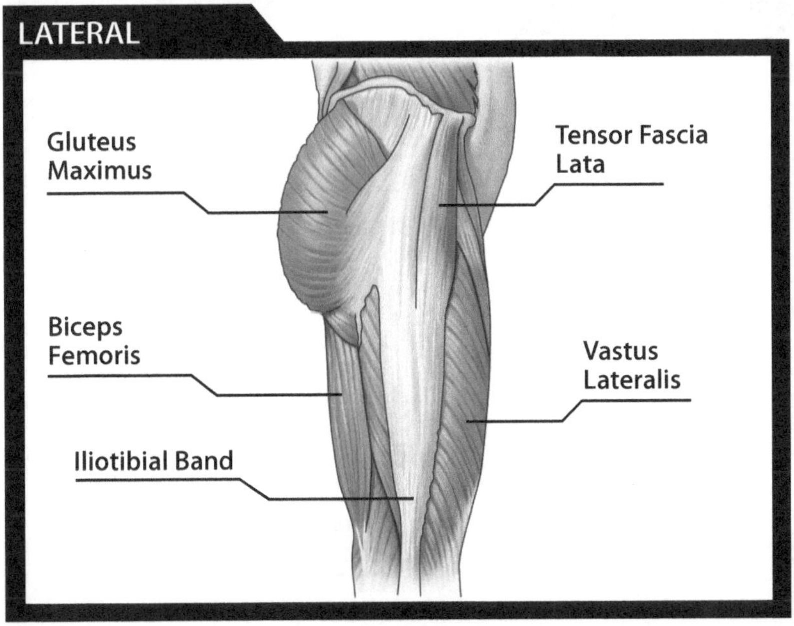

Anatomy Map: Pelvis

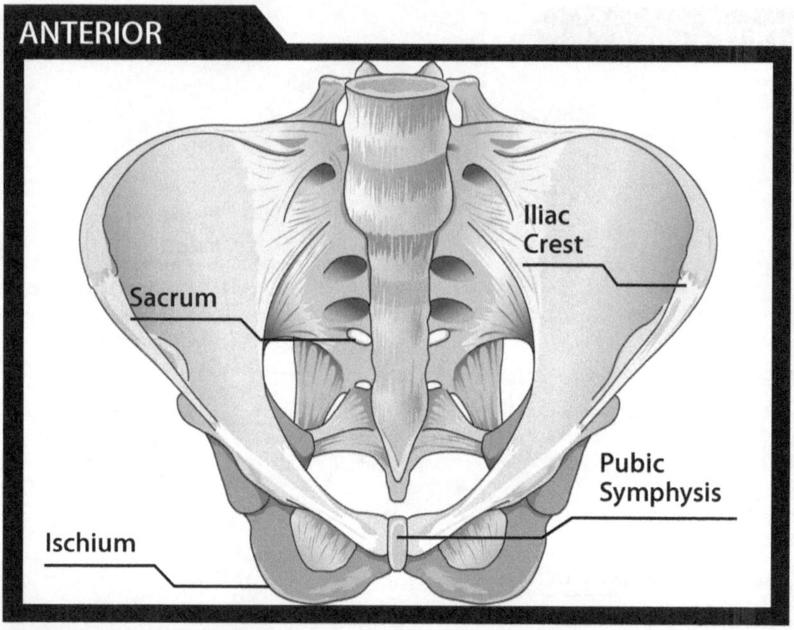

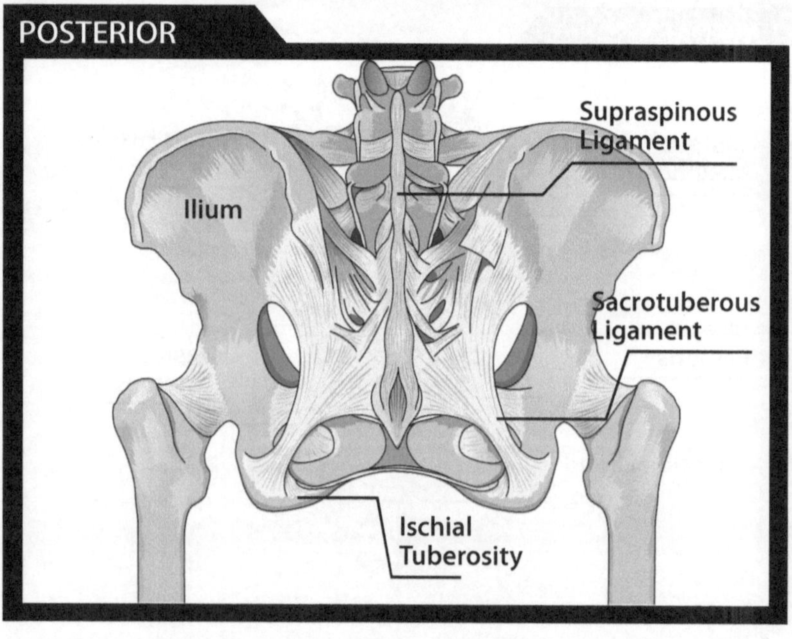

Anatomy Map: Pelvis

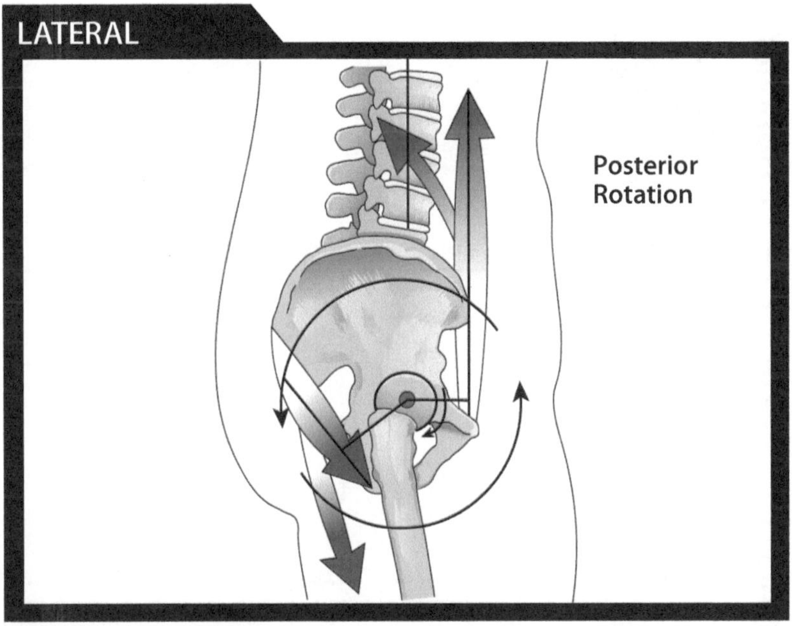

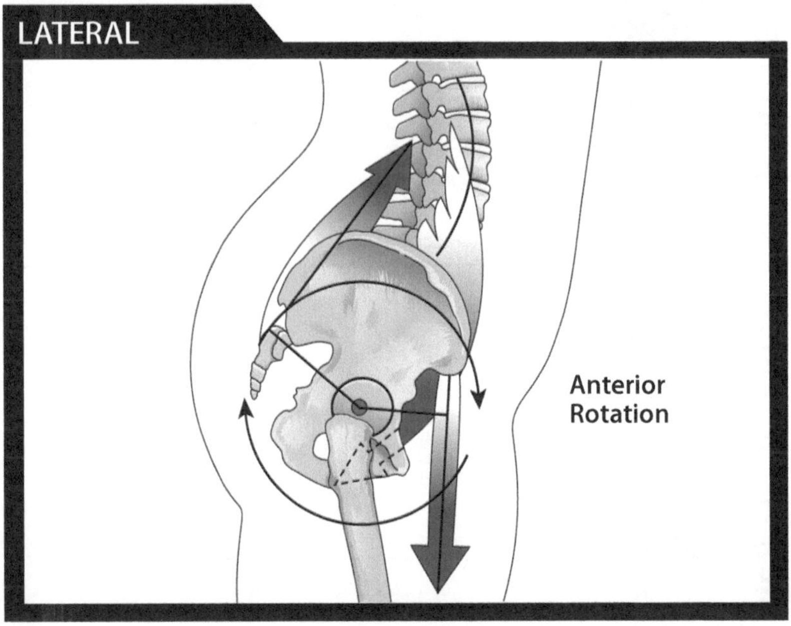

Hip/Thigh/Pelvis Pain Map: Region/Soft Tissue Differential Diagnosis

ANTERIOR

- Anterior Hip Dislocation
- Apophysitis
- Hip Flexor Strain
- Anterior Hip Impingement
- Quadriceps Contusion
- Quadriceps Strain
- Sartorius Strain
- Slipped Capital Femoral Epiphysis (SCFE)
- Snapping Hip Syndrome

POSTERIOR

- Ischial Bursitis
- Piriformis Syndrome
- Posterior Hip Dislocation
- Proximal Hamstring Avulsion
- Proximal Hamstring Strain
- Sciatica/Nerve Compression
- Sacroiliac (SI) Joint Dysfunction

MEDIAL

- Adductor Strain
- Labral Tear
- Osteitis Pubis*

**Refer to Osteitis Pubis versus Athletic Pubalgia (page 152)*

LATERAL

- Greater Trochanteric Bursitis
- Iliac Apophysitis

Hip/Thigh and Pelvis Pain

Injuries to Bone/Joint Surfaces

COMMON FRACTURES

- Pelvis
  - Acetabular
  - AIIS avulsion (rectus femoris)*
  - ASIS avulsion (sartorius)*
  - Ischial tuberosity avulsion (hamstring)*
  - Pubic rami avulsion (adductors)*
  - Pubic rami stress fracture
  - Sacral stress fracture
- Femur
  - Femoral head/neck (intracapsular)
  - Femoral neck stress fracture (compression/tension)
  - Femoral shaft stress fracture
  - Mid-proximal shaft of femur (extracapsular)

*Avulsion fractures are common in the skeletally immature patient. Clinicians must consider the possibility of an avulsion injury in this patient population.

Note: Stress fractures can result from mechanical loading factors and/or metabolic issues leading to insufficiency in bone health. Careful consideration must be given to patient history, activity level, and bone health. Suspicion of stress reaction to the femoral neck must be referred for appropriate follow up.

Clinical Assessment of Hip Injuries

Anterior Hip Pain

Anterior Hip Dislocation

HISTORY	MECHANISM OF INJURY	EVALUATION ESSENTIALS
• In athletic setting, hit from behind or fallen on with hip extended, adbducted, and externally rotated • Presents with possible deformity of hip position and leg length difference • Pain with and without weight bearing	• Traumatic force with hip in an extended, abducted, and externally rotated position	• Limited clinical exam • Palpation • Logical history • Diagnostic imaging is essential

KEY FINDINGS	DIAGNOSTIC EVIDENCE
• Clinical exam findings consistent with patient history • Evidence on radiographs • May be anterior-inferior or anterior-superior dislocation • Often associated with fractures to the femoral head (up to 75%) • This is a rare injury accounting for only 10% to 15% of all traumatic dislocations of the hip.	• Diagnostic imaging may require CT scans to fully evaluate femoral head • MRI is often used to determine extent of soft tissue injury[5]

Anterior Hip Pain

Apophysitis

HISTORY

- Patient reports pain at the apophysis (ASIS, AIIS, lesser trochanter)
- Patient may report swelling at apophysis
- Skeletally immature active patient

MECHANISM OF INJURY

- Repetitive jumping or running activities
- Forceful kicking

EVALUATION ESSENTIALS

- Palpation with possible palpable defect
- AROM and resisted range of motion (RROM) for involved muscle groups (pain and possible weakness)
- Diganostic imaging may be needed

KEY FINDINGS

- Clinical exam findings consistent with patient history
- In adolescents forceful movements and kicking can lead to avulsion fractures at the apophysis:
    - ASIS: sartorius
    - AIIS: rectus femoris
    - Lesser Trochanter: iliopsoas
- Careful MMT is essential

DIAGNOSTIC EVIDENCE

- Radiographs and MRI may used to evaluate possible avulsion injuries[6]

Anterior Hip/Thigh Pain

Hip Flexor Strain

HISTORY	MECHANISM OF INJURY	EVALUATION ESSENTIALS
• Sprinting, jumping, and landing activities • Patient reports anterior hip pain • Antalgic gait • Acute onset with possible popping sensation	• Acceleration to sprinting • Deceleration (eccentric load) from sprint • High velocity and high force movements at the hip • Sudden stop with hip and knee into flexion or an overstretch with hip in extension	• MMT of hip • AROM and PROM • Palpation of the hip flexor musculature

KEY FINDINGS	DIAGNOSTIC EVIDENCE
• Clinical exam findings consistent with patient history • Anterior hip pain reproduced with active testing • Pain with direct palpation • AROM reproduces pain • May not elicit pain with PROM	• Severe cases may warrant MRI evaluation to determine severity of injury and/or degree of tendon involvement • Diagnostic ultrasound is considered less sensitive than MRI and is user dependent[7] • MMT reliability: inter-rater (82% to 97%), intra-rater (96% to 98%)[8]

Anterior Hip Pain

Anterior Hip Impingement

HISTORY	MECHANISM OF INJURY	EVALUATION ESSENTIALS
• Anterior hip pain • Patient reports activities with repetitive hip flexion and rotation	• Repetitive hip flexion with rotation • Cam (femoral) or pincer (acetabulum) bony deformity • High velocity and high force movements at the hip	• FADIR (flexion, adduction, internal rotation) test • Hip scouring test

KEY FINDINGS	DIAGNOSTIC EVIDENCE
• Also called femoral acetabular impingement • Clinical exam findings consistent with patient history • Anterior hip pain with FADIR • Anterior hip pain with hip scouring test • Pain with both active and passive hip flexion with rotation if cam or pincer deformity present	• Radiographs to evaluate cam and pincer deformities • Estimated prevalence is 10% to 15% of the population • Cam more common in men; pincer more common in women[9]

Anterior Hip/Thigh Pain

Quadriceps Contusion

HISTORY	MECHANISM OF INJURY	EVALUATION ESSENTIALS
• Patient presents with pain and loss of function following a direct blow • Patient describes loss of function and pain with muscle activation • Antalgic gait	• Direct blow to the anterior thigh	• Palpation of the quadriceps • AROM and PROM • MMT of thigh (knee flexion)

KEY FINDINGS	DIAGNOSTIC EVIDENCE
• Clinical exam findings consistent with patient history • Correlation of history with direct palpation • Ecchymosis and possible edema	• Imaging may be warranted if myositis ossificans complication is suspected[10]

Anterior Hip/Thigh Pain

Quadriceps Strain

HISTORY	MECHANISM OF INJURY	EVALUATION ESSENTIALS
• Sprinting, jumping, and landing activities • Patient reports anterior hip/thigh pain • May present with loss of knee flexion and muscle tightness • Antalgic gait • Acute onset with possible popping sensation • Possible defect	• Acceleration to sprinting • Deceleration (eccentric load) from sprint • High velocity and high force movements at the hip and thigh • Sudden stop with hip and knee into flexion or an overstretch with hip in extension	• MMT of thigh (knee flexion) • AROM and PROM • Palpation of the quadriceps

KEY FINDINGS	DIAGNOSTIC EVIDENCE
• Clinical exam findings consistent with patient history • Anterior thigh pain reproduced with active testing • Pain with direct palpation • Contract the quadriceps and palpate for defect to aid in determining degree of injury	• Severe cases may warrant MRI evaluation to determine severity of injury and/or degree of tendon involvement • Diagnostic ultrasound is considered less sensitive than MRI and is user dependent[7] • MMT reliability: inter-rater (82% to 97%), intra-rater (96% to 98%)[8]

Anterior Hip/Thigh Pain

Sartorius Strain

HISTORY	MECHANISM OF INJURY	EVALUATION ESSENTIALS
• Sprinting, jumping, and landing activities • Patient reports anterior hip/thigh pain • Antalgic gait is possible • Patient reports loss of knee and hip flexion • Possible swelling	• Acceleration and deceleration (eccentric load) activities • High velocity and high force movements at the hip and thigh • Sudden stop with hip and knee into flexion with external rotation or an overstretch with hip in extension	• MMT of the sartorius: hip flexion with hip external rotation • AROM and PROM at the hip

KEY FINDINGS	DIAGNOSTIC EVIDENCE
• Clinical exam findings consistent with patient history • Pain reproduced with active testing of hip flexion and external rotation	• Severe cases may warrant MRI evaluation to determine severity of injury and/or degree of tendon involvement • Diagnostic ultrasound is considered less sensitive than MRI and is user dependent[7] • MMT reliability: inter-rater (82% to 97%), intra-rater (96% to 98%)[8]

Anterior Hip/Thigh Pain

Slipped Capital Femoral Epiphysis

HISTORY	MECHANISM OF INJURY	EVALUATION ESSENTIALS
• Patient reports groin pain as a result of trauma or over weeks or months as a result of prolonged stress • Pain with active and passive motion • Limitation in abduction, flexion, and internal rotation • Antalgic gait	• Trauma or prolonged stress	• Complete and thorough hip evaluation is essential • MMT of the hip • AROM and PROM at the hip • Long axis hip pressure/scouring

KEY FINDINGS	DIAGNOSTIC EVIDENCE
• Clinical exam findings consistent with patient history • Essential to listen closely to the history and suggest images for full evaluation; low tolerance to refer for radiograph if history suggests SCFE • SCFEs are mostly found in boys ages 10 to 17 that are either tall and thin or obese; can be bilateral	• Radiographic imaging is essential to idenfity a SCFE[11]

Anterior Hip/Thigh Pain

Snapping Hip Syndrome

HISTORY	MECHANISM OF INJURY	EVALUATION ESSENTIALS
• Patient reports audible popping, or clicking in the anterior hip region with activity • Clicking or popping may or may not involve pain	• Overuse injury that presents with repeated flexion and sometimes external rotation maneuvers	• Thorough evaluation to rule out hip joint pain and pathology • AROM and PROM at the hip • MMT of the hip • Clinician should reproduce hip flexion with external rotation to reproduce symptoms

KEY FINDINGS	DIAGNOSTIC EVIDENCE
• Clinical exam findings consistent with patient history • Complete exam is warranted since snapping hip may be confused with greater trochanteric bursitis, intra-articular loose body, or labral tear • Audible pop or click with hip flexion and/or with external rotation	• Diagnosed by clinical exam and ruling out of other pathology • No diagnostic evidence available

Posterior Hip Pain

Ischial Bursitis

HISTORY	MECHANISM OF INJURY	EVALUATION ESSENTIALS
• Patient reports pain in the buttock, particularly with sitting on a hard surface • Pain with hamstring contraction • Pain with high force production and attenuation	• Repetitive or prolonged activity (eg, running, kicking, or jumping) • Can occur with trauma by falling on a hard surface	• TTP over palpable tenderness over the ischial bursa • Imaging may be needed • MMT

KEY FINDINGS	DIAGNOSTIC EVIDENCE
• Clinical exam findings consistent with patient history • Pain with sitting • Pain from the friction of bursa from the hamstring tendon	• Severe cases may warrant diagnostic imaging • Ultrasound imaging, CT scan, or MRI • Radiographs to rule out bony involvement[12]

Posterior Hip Pain

Piriformis Syndrome

HISTORY	MECHANISM OF INJURY	EVALUATION ESSENTIALS
• Pain in the buttock that may or may not radiate • May have numbness or tingling in buttock or posterior thigh • Possible history of trauma • May report participation in a repetitive activity or prolonged sitting	• Prolonged sitting • Repetitive activities (eg, running or lunging)	• Piriformis MMT • TTP over the piriformis • Piriformis test for soft tissue immobility • MRI can be used for definitive testing

KEY FINDINGS	DIAGNOSTIC EVIDENCE
• Clinical exam findings consistent with patient history • This can be a diagnosis of exclusion • Presence of numbness and tingling warrants differntial diagnosis with discogenic pathologies	• Sciatic nerve pain has a lifetime prevalence of 12.2% to 27% in the general population; it is unclear how many of these cases are due to piriformis syndrome • The piriformis test on its own has shown variable results in the literature[13]

Posterior Hip Pain

Posterior Hip Dislocation

HISTORY	MECHANISM OF INJURY	EVALUATION ESSENTIALS
• Patient reports pain and sense of deformity in the hip • Possible numbness and tingling	• Explosive sprinting, jumping, and landing activities • Rapid acceleration or deceleration movements • Eccentric load on muscle tissue • Hip is vulnerable to dislocation in the hip flexion, adduction, and internal rotation position	• Palpation and imaging are best for accurate diagnosis • Do not pursue active or passive motions of the hip

KEY FINDINGS	DIAGNOSTIC EVIDENCE
• If hip dislocation is suspected, patient needs to be transported to a care facility for imaging and joint reduction • Affected extremity will appear shorter and internally rotated • This injury is common in adolescents and following hip joint replacement surgery	• Following hip replacement surgery, approximately 9% of patients experience a posterior hip dislocation[14]

Posterior Hip Pain

Proximal Hamstring Avulsion

HISTORY	MECHANISM OF INJURY	EVALUATION ESSENTIALS
• Patient reports history of popping in the buttock region associated with MOI • Explosive activity (eg, jumping, landing, sprinting)	• Explosive sprinting, jumping, and landing activities • Rapid acceleration or deceleration movements • Eccentric load on muscle tissue	• TTP over the ischial tuberosity • Palpable deformity • MMT

KEY FINDINGS	DIAGNOSTIC EVIDENCE
• Clinical exam findings consistent with patient history • Patient may hear "pop" or feel sensation of popping • True avulsion of the hamstring is rare • The ischial apophysis closes in the late teens to early 20s	• Severe cases may warrant MRI evaluation to determine severity of injury[15]

Posterior Hip Pain

Proximal Hamstring Strain

HISTORY	MECHANISM OF INJURY	EVALUATION ESSENTIALS
• Patient reports an acute onset of injury • Patient describes pain in the buttocks region • Ecchymosis depending upon the severity of strain	• Explosive sprinting, jumping, and landing activities • Rapid acceleration or deceleration movements • Eccentric load on muscle tissue	• TTP over the ischial tuberosity, swelling • MMT for each specific hamstring • 90-degree versus 15-degree testing to differentiate hip extension and knee flexion

KEY FINDINGS	DIAGNOSTIC EVIDENCE
• Grades 1 to 3 with 3 being full rupture • Symptoms vary depending upon the level of strain • Clinical exam findings consistent with patient history • Severe strain typically does not result in audible pop like avulsion injury • Rapid onset of pain • Loss of function	• MRI can be used for severe injuries (sensitivity 33% to 100%, specificity 92% to 100%) • Diagnostic ultrasound for muscle strain evaluation (sensitivity 79% to 100%, specificity 92%)[16] • Predisposing factors include: increased age, previous hamstring injury, fatigue, decreased flexibility, and muscle imbalance[17]

Posterior Hip Pain

Sciatica/Nerve Compression

HISTORY	MECHANISM OF INJURY	EVALUATION ESSENTIALS
• Pain in the buttock radiating down the leg • Repetitive activity • Patient may report low back discomfort • Abrupt or gradual discomfort • Sharp shooting pain that follows the nerve root • May have numbness or tingling	• Repetitive activity • Participation in a unilateral sport activity for a long duration	• Straight leg raise (SLR) test (30 to 60 degrees) • Bowstring test

KEY FINDINGS	DIAGNOSTIC EVIDENCE
• Clinical exam findings consistent with patient history • Sciatica is a symptom and not a condition in and of itself which is why we describe this condition as "nerve compression" • Presence of numbness and tingling warrants differntial diagnosis with discogenic pathologies	• SLR validity and reliability is highly variable among the literature due to confounding factors such as age, source of pain, and patient positioning • Bowstring test validity and reliability is unreported in the literature[18]

Posterior Hip Pain

Sacroiliac Joint Dysfunction

HISTORY	MECHANISM OF INJURY	EVALUATION ESSENTIALS
• Patient may report low back and posterior hip or buttock pain • May point to the SI joint as area of tenderness • Reports increased pain in SI with weight shift to one leg and/or unilateral stance	• Repetitive activity unilateral • Over rotating with a particular sport activity (eg, golf, dance, punting, high jumping, hurdling, or gymnastics)	• SI compression, distraction, and pelvic tilt • Gillet's, forward flexion test • Seated sacral flexion and extension tests • FABER test • SLR testing (70 to 90 degrees) • ASIS and PSIS symmetry

KEY FINDINGS	DIAGNOSTIC EVIDENCE
• Clinical exam findings consistent with patient history • Must have multiple positive tests to diagnose true SI dysfunction[19]	• Compression test (sensitivity 63%, specificity 69%) • Distraction test (sensitivity 60%, specificity 81%) • FABER test (sensitivity 63%, specificity 76%) • Gillet's test (sensitivity 43%, specificity 68%)[20]

Medial Hip Pain

Adductor Strain

HISTORY	MECHANISM OF INJURY	EVALUATION ESSENTIALS
• Patient reports an acute onset of pain • Possible swelling • Loss of hip abduction • Pain with hip flexion • Loss of soft tissue mobility • Antalgic gait	• Overstretch with hip in abduction • Jumping or twisting MOI • Overuse with hip external rotation	• Adductor MMT • Hip flexor MMT

KEY FINDINGS	DIAGNOSTIC EVIDENCE
• Grades 1 to 3 with 3 being full rupture • Symptoms vary with severity • Clinical exam findings consistent with patient history • Pain location • MMT consistent with history and palpation findings • The groin is common area of referred pain; must rule out other pain sources (eg, osteoarthritis of the hip and back pain)	• Severe cases may warrant MRI evaluation to determine severity of injury and/or degree of tendon involvement • Diagnostic ultrasound is considered less sensitive than MRI and is user dependent[7] • MMT reliability: inter-rater (82% to 97%), intra-rater (96% to 98%)[8]

Medial Hip Pain

Labral Tear

HISTORY	MECHANISM OF INJURY	EVALUATION ESSENTIALS
• May also present as anterior hip pain • Mechanical symptoms (eg, catching) • Locking of hip joint • Patient describes pain at hip radiating to thigh when going from sitting to standing • Possible groin or lower abdominal pain	• Direct trauma • Twisting injury into external rotation • Repetitive motions (eg, rotation, hyperextension, and abduction)	• Hip scouring • AROM and PROM • MRI or CT scan

KEY FINDINGS	DIAGNOSTIC EVIDENCE
• Clinical exam findings consistent with patient history • Pain location • Pain with hip scouring • The groin and hip are common areas of referred pain; must rule out other pain sources (eg, osteoarthritis of the hip and back pain)	• Hip scour (sensitivity 75% to 89%, specificity 15% to 43%) • MRI (sensitivity 25% to 30%) • Magnetic resonance arthrogram (MRA) (sensitivity 66% to 90%) • CT (sensitivity 92% to 97%, specificity 87% to 100%)[21,22]

Lateral Hip Pain

Greater Trochanteric Bursitis

HISTORY	MECHANISM OF INJURY	EVALUATION ESSENTIALS
• Pain with hip motions • Patient can't lie on the affected side • Antalgic gait • Loss of motion	• Direct blow trauma • Overuse and repetivie motion	• Palpation of the greater trochanteric bursa • MMT • Ober's test for the iliotibial band

KEY FINDINGS	DIAGNOSTIC EVIDENCE
• Clinical exam findings consistent with patient history • Patient experiences tenderness over the greater trochanter • Postivie Ober's test	• Sensitivity and specificity of Ober's test is not cited in the literature but is often positive • Anesthetic injection of the bursa can be used as a diagnostic and therapeutic tool • MRI and ultrasound may be used to determine if there are other contributing factors in the hip, pelvis, or low back[23]

Lateral Hip Pain

Iliac Apophysitis

HISTORY	MECHANISM OF INJURY	EVALUATION ESSENTIALS
• Patient describes localized pain and swelling at the iliac crest • Pain increases with use of the muscles that attach at the iliac crest	• Repetitive jumping or running activities • Rapid increase in work load or work volume	• Palpation of iliac apophysis • Radiographic imaging • MMT

KEY FINDINGS	DIAGNOSTIC EVIDENCE
• Clinical exam findings consistent with patient history • Common in adolescents • Can lead to avulsion fractures	• Radiographs are often inconclusive, but widening of the physis can be seen with the use of MRI[23]

Osteitis Pubis versus Athletic Pubalgia

CONSIDERATIONS FOR EVALUATION

- Overview
    - Clinicians must be aware of these overuse conditions that can cause lower abdominal, groin, and pubic symphysis discomfort in the active patient. The diagnosis and subsequent care of these injuries can be difficult as many symptoms and clinical findings overlap. Confusion over the ultimate cause of patient pain can lead to a delayed diagnosis and prolonged pain and dysfunction. In addition, the nomenclature can contribute to the confusion as *athletic pubalgia* is sometimes used interchangeably with the term *sports hernia.*
- Similarities
    - Patients with both of these conditions tend to present with pain in the central pubic region, both occur due to repetitive stress at the pubic symphysis region, and unilateral stress from kicking as one cause. These injuries are common in soccer, ice hockey, football, and other sports that require strong core control of the muscles around the pubic bone. Patients with either problem may be point tender at the pubic tubercle.
- Differences
    - *Osteitis pubis:* pain may originate in the groin initially and progress to tenderness over the pubic tubercle. Pain with running, doing sit ups, and squats.
    - *Athletic pubalgia:* pain starts in the lower abdomen and inguinal region, progressing to the adductors and testicles in males. Pain increased with resisted hip flexion, internal rotation and abdominal muscle contraction. Pain also with resisted hip adduction and adductors are not tender to palpation.

Sacroiliac Joint Dysfunction

INNOMINATE ROTATION AND MALALIGNMENT

SACROILIAC JOINT DYSFUNCTION

Sacroiliac joint dysfunction (SIJD) is likely caused by a change in how the right and left sacroiliac joints work together. If there is too much (hypermobility) or too little (hypomobility) between the right and left innominate bones the result will be a pelvic obliquity. In normal alignment the innominate bones are in equal position. During SIJD one side may present in a variety of dysfunctional alignments (anterior rotation, posterior rotation, etc) causing SI joint pain.

COMMON SIJD ALIGNMENTS

- *Anterior/posterior innominate*: anterior or posterior rotation of the ilium on one side. ASIS and PSIS on one side will be higher and lower, or lower and higher, respectively; utilize SI testing to assess this along with supine to sit test leg length test.
- *Upslip/downslip*: unilateral elevation or depression of the ilium. Evaluate the iliac crest and ischial tuberosity on the side of pain and/or injury.
- *Inflare/outflare*: unilateral rotation (in or out) of the ilium on the sacrum. This is evaluated by examining the position of the ASIS and PSIS (medial or lateral alignment).
- Sacral torsions: rotation or torsion of the sacrum around a diagnonal axis. One side or pole of the sacrum is prominent by comparison.
    - Torsion positions: left on left, right on right, left on right, right on left
    - Assess in sacral flexion and extension, palpate the sacral bases and inferior lateral angles (ILAs)
- SIJDs present a diagnostic challenge and require significant clinical practice to become proficient. Improving these assessment techniques may require clinicians to pursue additional continuing education.

Paper Patient: Revisited

You should have been able to rule out several conditions secondary to knowing what structures are at the anterior hip. Your differential should have been snapping hip syndrome versus labral tear.

Learning Activities: Practice Case

Use the blank templates provided in the Appendices to write out a differential diagnosis map and clinical findings overview for the case provided below. When working with paper patients, it is tempting to try to jump to "the answer" and come to a diagnosis. However, the visual learning approach to differential diagnosis is designed to help you consider all the possibilities for the information provided. Good luck.

Paper Patient: Anterior Hip Pain in a Middle-aged Female

History

Julie is a 47-year-old female who presents to you with a chief complaint of left anterior hip pain. The worst activity for her is putting on her underwear. She walks everywhere for activity, as well as going to boot camp classes. She will have pain after cleaning the bathroom. She has had to cut down on her exercise because the pain has been getting worse. She can't sleep on the right side because of pain on the left. She reports that she has had hip pain on and off for about 10 years, and last year she was diagnosed with SIJD and was given exercises that were helpful. She has tried to do the exercises again, but this time they are not helping. She is getting popping in her hip that is scaring her. She feels like she needs to readjust her hip by pulling it backward so she can do what she needs to do. The pain moves into her groin sometimes as well.

Physical Exam

Her physical exam reveals diffuse tenderness to palpation at the hip. Her MMT demonstrated weakness in the gluteals, hamstrings, and hip external rotators. There is pain with passive motion; active hip flexion produces pain as well. FABER and FADIR tests were positive, and hip scouring was negative. Active hip internal rotation and external rotation were measured with a goniometer and recorded as 22 degrees and 20 degrees on the left, respectively, and 26 degrees and 24 degrees on the right, respectively.

References

1. Keogh MJ, Batt ME. A review of femoroacetabular impingement in athletes. *Sports Med.* 2008;38(10):863-878.
2. Moeller JL. Pelvic and hip apophyseal avulsion injuries in young athletes. *Curr Sports Med Rep.* 2003;2(2):110-115.
3. Powell JW, Barber-Foss KD. Injury patterns in selected high school sports: A review of the 1995-1997 seasons. *J Athl Train.* 1999;34(3):277.
4. Agel J. Descriptive epidemiology of collegiate men's soccer injuries: National Collegiate Athletic Association Injury Surveillance System, 1988–1989 through 2002–2003. *J Athl Train.* 2007;42(2):270.
5. Pallia CS, Scott RE, Chao DJ. Traumatic hip dislocation in athletes. *Curr Sports Med Rep.* 2002;1(6):338-345.
6. Arnaiz J, Piedra T, de Lucas EM, et al. Imaging findings of lower limb apophysitis. *AJR Am J Roentgenol.* 2011;196(3):W316-325.
7. Hayashi D, Hamilton B, Guermazi A, de Villiers R, Crema MD, Roemer FW. Traumatic injuries of thigh and calf muscles in athletes: Role and clinical relevance of MR imaging and ultrasound. *Insights Imaging.* 2012;3(6):591-601.
8. Cuthbert SC, Goodheart GJ Jr. On the reliability and validity of manual muscle testing: A literature review. *Chiropr Osteopat.* 2007;15:4.
9. Ochoa LM, Dawson L, Patzkowski JC, Hsu JR. Radiographic prevalence of femoracetabular impingement in a young population with hip complaints is high. *Clin Orthop Relat Res.* 2010;468(10):2710-2714.
10. Kary JM. Diagnosis and management of quadriceps strains and contusions. *Curr Rev Musculoskelet Med.* 2010;3(1-4):26-31.
11. Jarrett DY, Matheney T, Kleinman PK. Imaging SCFE: Diagnosis, treatment and complications. *Pediatr Radiol.* 2013;43(Suppl 1):S71-82.
12. Paluska SA. An overview of hip injuries in running. Sports Med. 2005;35(11):991-1014.
13. Hopayian K, Song F, Riera R, Sambandan S. The clinical features of the piriformis syndrome: A systematic review. *Eur Spine J.* 2010;19(12):2095-2109.
14. Burgers PT, Van Geene AR, Van den Bekerom MP, et al. Total hip arthroplasty versus hemiarthroplasty for displaced femoral neck fractures in the healthy elderly: A meta-analysis and systematic review of randomized trials. *Int Orthop.* 2012;36(8):1549-1560.
15. Koulouris G, Connell D. Evaluation of the hamstring muscle complex following acute injury. *Skeletal Radiol.* 2003;32(10):582-589.
16. Hodgson RJ, O'Connor PJ, Grainger AJ. Tendon and ligament imaging. *Br J Radiol.* 2012;85(1016):1157-1172.
17. Heiderscheit BC, Sherry MA, Silder A, Chumanov ES, Thelen DG. Hamstring strain injuries: Recommendations for diagnosis, rehabilitation, and injury prevention. *J Orthop Sports Phys Ther.* 2010;40(2):67-81.
18. van der Windt DA, Simons E, Riphagen II, et al. Physical examination for lumbar radiculopathy due to disc herniation in patients with low-back pain. *Cochrane Database Syst Rev.* 2010;17(2):CD007431.
19. Riddle D, Freburger J. Evaluation of the Presence of Sacroiliac Joint Region Dysfunction Using a Combination of Tests: A Multicenter Intertester Reliability Study. *Physical Therapy* [serial online]. 2002;82(8):772-781.
20. Szadek KM, van der Wurff P, van Tulder MW, Zuurmond WW, Perez RS. Diagnostic validity of criteria for sacroiliac joint pain: A systematic review. *J Pain.* 2009;10(4):354-368.

21. Tijssen M, van Cingel R, Willemsen L, de Visser E. Diagnostics of femoroacetabular impingement and labral pathology of the hip: A systematic review of the accuracy and validity of physical tests. *Arthroscopy.* 2012;28(6):860-867.
22. Burgess RM, Rushton A, Wright C, Daborn C. The validity and accuracy of clinical diagnostic tests used to detect labral pathology of the hip: A systematic review. *Man Ther.* 2011;16(4):318-326.
23. Strauss EJ, Nho SJ, Kelly BT. Greater trochanteric pain syndrome. *Sports Med Arthrosc.* 2010;18(2):113-119.
24. Hébert KJ, Laor T, Divine JG, Emery KH, Wall EJ. MRI appearance of chronic stress injury of the iliac crest apophysis in adolescent athletes. *AJR Am J Roentgenol.* 2008;190(6):1487-1491.

6

The Spine

Low back pain is the fifth most common reason for seeking medical care in the United States.[1] Carey et al[2] reported that 25% of all adults in the United States report having low back pain at least once a day in the past 3 months, and 7.6% report at least one episode of acute back pain within the past year. The prevalence rate of low back pain in athletes (1% to 40%) varies greatly by sport activity. Trainor[3] found that athletes participating in gymnastics, diving, weight lifting, golf, American football, and rowing have shown higher rates of back pain. Also, 90% of the injuries sustained by professional golfers involve the neck and back. The back injury rate in gymnastics is over 10%, and back pain in American football linemen has been reported as high as 50%.[4] Auvinen et al[5] found injury rates for adolescent girls in gymnastics, dance, or physical education are higher than the general population, while cross-country skiing and aerobics are associated with a lower prevalence of low back pain. For boys, volleyball, gymnastics, weight lifting, downhill skiing, and snowboarding are associated with higher prevalence of low back pain, while cross-country skiing and aerobics show a lower prevalence.

It is important for clinicians to remember that back pain is a symptom that has many underlying causes. An et al[6] reported that muscle strains, ligament sprains, and soft tissue contusions account for over 95% of back pain in the general adult population. The majority of athletes with low back pain have nonpathological sources of pain,[7] and muscle strain may be the most common cause of low back pain in college athletes.[8] Micheli and

Winterstein AP, Clark SV. *The Athletic Trainer's Guide to Differential Diagnosis (pp 157-202).*

Wood[9] reported that repetitive extension injuries (eg, gymnastics, figure skating, diving, and football linemen) along the spectrum of spondylolysis to spondylolisthesis are identified as the most common cause of low back pain in adolescents. Bono[10] reported the prevalence of radiographic evidence of disc degeneration is higher in athletes than it is in nonathletes; however, it remains unclear whether this correlates with a higher rate of back pain. Most episodes of low back pain are short-lived, and 80% to 90% of attacks of low back pain resolve in about 6 weeks, regardless of treatment. However, multiple studies in the late 90s showed recurrent or chronic low back pain evaluated at 3, 6, or 12 months, and recurrence or persistence of pain ranged from 35% to 79%.[11]

Petering and Webb[12] emphasized that the clinical examination and diagnostic skills are essential in the workup of low back pain, and the workup and diagnosis must be individualized on the basis of differential diagnosis. The differential diagnosis maps provided in this chapter differ from our other regional maps in that they divide the injury possibilities into central, peripheral, and radiating classifications. While the lumbar region will be the most common of the spine evaluations, clinicians must be prepared to assess injuries to the thoracic and cervical spine as well. This chapter presents differential diagnosis maps and clinical findings for all three regions of the spine.

Paper Patient: Low Back Pain in a Swimmer

History

Ben is a 14-year-old swimmer, soccer player, and runner who complains of back pain. He reports that he has grown quite a bit from the spring into the summer. He participated in summer swimming and his strokes are freestyle and breaststroke. He plays soccer year round (outdoor in fall and spring and indoor in winter). He likes running and is planning to join cross-country in the fall. He started the weight training class over the summer with his friends and then he was training with the other cross-country runners three times per week. The weight training involved heavy squats and hang cleans with just a bit more than his body weight. You discover that he did not have instruction on lifting from anyone—he just did what his friends were doing.

Physical Exam

Your exam reveals tenderness to palpation over the spinous processes at L5 and over the paraspinals starting in the mid portion of the thoracic spine. The patient has pain with active motion from deep flexion to extension bilaterally, lateral flexion bilaterally, and rotation bilaterally. You feel a step off at L5 to S1 on palpation. Hamstring testing in the 90/90 position was positive for tightness bilaterally. The patient has hip flexor tightness as measured prone and in the Thomas test position. There is palpable spasm along the paraspinals from the upper lumbar into mid thoracic region. There is a positive stork stance test.

Using the information from your clinical exam, ask yourself these questions to guide your clinical decision making:

- What is your differential diagnosis?
- What key findings do you see to help guide your differential?
- What are the possible injuries associated with these findings?

Clinical Decisions

Start with a review of the anatomy maps and a thorough consideration of the possible injuries and conditions that are common to the spine. Use the differential diagnosis maps to guide your thought process and organize the possibilities. The organized synthesis of this information is the essence of clinical decision making. We will revisit this case at the end of the chapter.

Anatomy Map: Knee

ANTERIOR

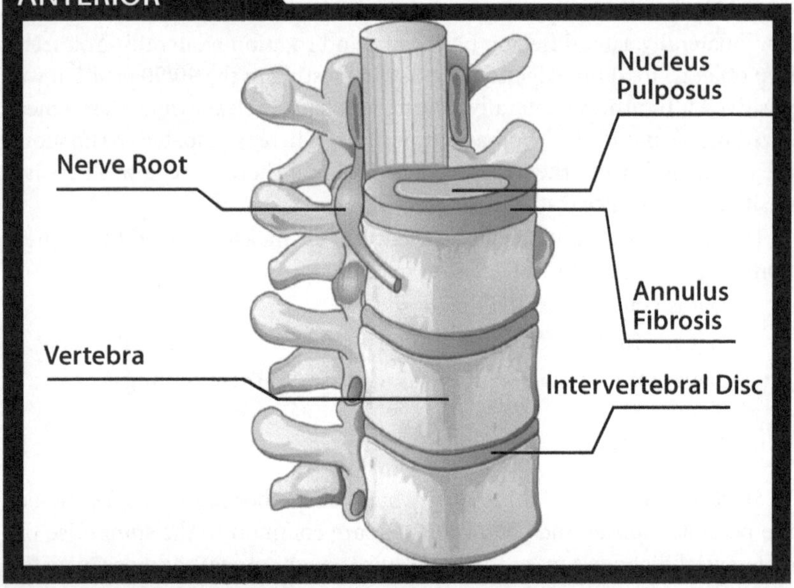

LATERAL

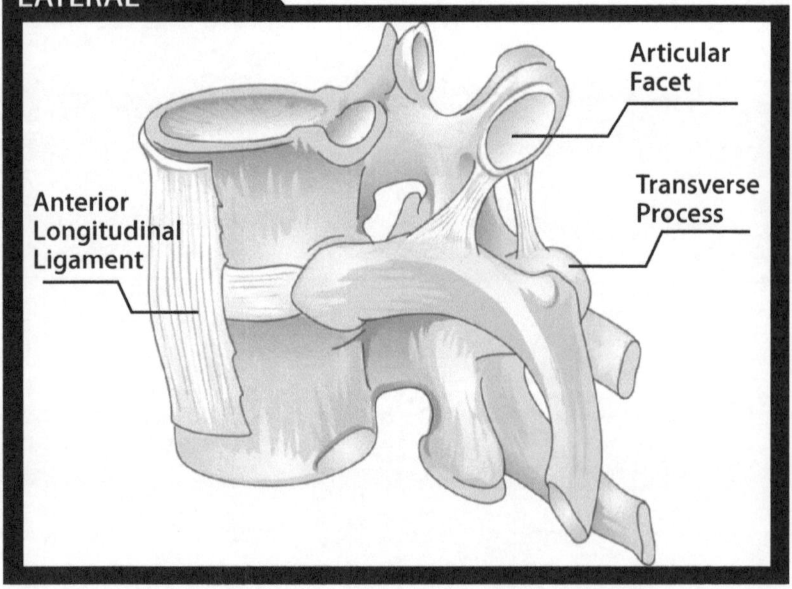

Anatomy Map: Knee

LATERAL

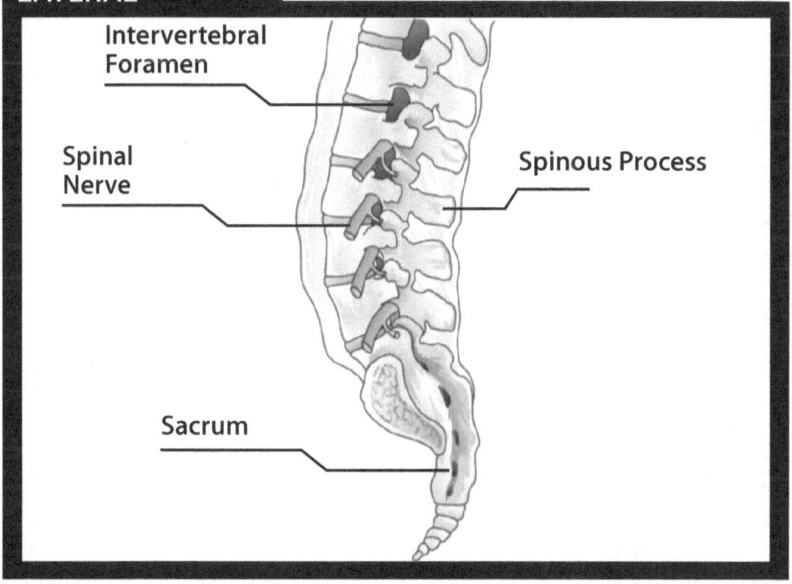

POSTERIOR

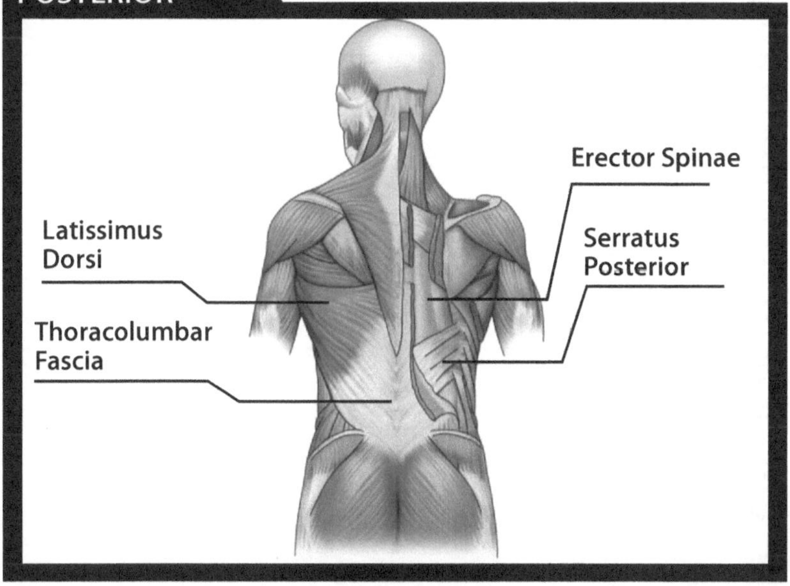

Cervical Spine: Region/Soft Tissue Differential Diagnosis

CENTRAL

- Cervical Sprain/Strain
- Facet Joint Dysfunction
- Intervertebral Disc Lesion/Herniation

PERIPHERAL

- Paraspinal Strain/Spasm
- Scalene Strain/Spasm
- Upper Trapezius Strain/Spasm

RADIATING/DISTAL

- Brachial Plexus Injury
- Cervical Cord Injury
- Cervical Spondylosis
- Intervertebral Disc Lesion/Herniation
- Nerve Root Impingement

Clinical Assessment of Cervical Spine Injuries

Central Cervical Spine Pain

Cervical Sprain/Strain

HISTORY	MECHANISM OF INJURY	EVALUATION ESSENTIALS
• Patient reports a sudden force either by contact or acceleration or deceleration like a whiplash • Acute onset • Pain identified with motion at the neck	• Sudden muscular contractions trying to decelerate head • Forced cervical rotation • Sprains and strains occur together, posterior muscles are strained resisting flexion, and anterior strained resisting hyperextension	• Assess tenderness to palpation • Inspect for swelling • Evaluate muscle strength

KEY FINDINGS	DIAGNOSTIC EVIDENCE
• The patient will have pain and swelling either anterior or posterior depending upon the mechanism • The patient will have a history of head contact with an opponent or ground or whiplash injury	• Dynamic radiographs may be taken to determine if ligamentous laxity has caused cervical instability[13]

Central Cervical Spine Pain

Facet Joint Dysfunction

HISTORY	MECHANISM OF INJURY	EVALUATION ESSENTIALS
• Patient reports restricted motion and pain • Chronic or acute onset • Pain identified with rotation, extension, and/or lateral flexion	• Osteoarthritis • Trauma • Posture • Sudden twist or whiplash	• Palpation of the cervical spine • Assess cervical extension, flexion, lateral flexion, and rotation • Evaluate mobility of facets

KEY FINDINGS	DIAGNOSTIC EVIDENCE
• The patient will have pain in the posterior neck to the shoulder; no radicular symptoms • The patient likely will have history of extension, quick movement, sleeping with neck hanging to one side, or twisting movement • The patient will have a facet that has become hypomobile	• No diagnostic evidence available

Central Cervical Spine Pain

Intervertebral Disc Lesion/Herniation

HISTORY	MECHANISM OF INJURY	EVALUATION ESSENTIALS
• Patient reports neck pain, numbness and tingling, or radicular pain • Chronic or acute onset	• Trauma • Sustained, repetitive cervical loading during contact sports • Degenerative changes from wear and tear on the disc over time	• Assess AROM and PROM • Inspect cervical spine through palpation • Cervical compression, shoulder abduction test, and Spurling's test • Evaluate muscle strength

KEY FINDINGS	DIAGNOSTIC EVIDENCE
• The patient will have pain in the neck and decreased ROM • The patient may complain of numbness and tingling, radicular pain, and quadriparesis	• MRI may be used to confirm the diagnosis • Spurling's test (sensitivity 92%, specificity 95%)[14]

Peripheral Cervical Spine Pain

Paraspinal Strain/Spasm

HISTORY	MECHANISM OF INJURY	EVALUATION ESSENTIALS
• Patient reports neck pain either unilateral or bilateral • Chronic or acute onset • Pain identified with active extension	• Sudden extension contraction on an overloaded, unprepared, or underdeveloped spine in combination with trunk rotation • Poor posture	• Assess active and passive cervical range of motion • Palpate paraspinal muscles • Evaluate muscle strength

KEY FINDINGS	DIAGNOSTIC EVIDENCE
• The patient will have either local or diffuse pain • The pain will be with active extension and passive flexion • There will be no radiating or neurological symptoms	• No diagnostic evidence available

Peripheral Cervical Spine Pain

Scalene Strain/Spasm

HISTORY	MECHANISM OF INJURY	EVALUATION ESSENTIALS
• Patient reports neck and arm pain • Chronic onset • Pain identified with stretching or compression of the scalenes	• Chronic muscle overuse • Poor posture • Repetitive micro trauma to muscle	• Assess AROM and PROM • Inspect scalenes for trigger points • TOS testing, cervical radiculopathy testing • Evaluate muscle strength of the scalenes

KEY FINDINGS	DIAGNOSTIC EVIDENCE
• This mimics cervical TOS pathology • The radiating symptoms down the arm will typically be in the C6 nerve root distribution • The patient will likely have trigger points that reproduce symptoms when palpated • Often misdiagnosed as cervical pathology	• No diagnostic evidence available

Peripheral Cervical Spine Pain

Upper Trapezius Strain/Spasm

HISTORY	MECHANISM OF INJURY	EVALUATION ESSENTIALS
• Patient reports headache and pain in neck and shoulder • Chronic or acute onset • Pain identified with motion after resting	• Overloading the muscle • Poor posture • Overusing muscle • Stress	• Assess posture • Inspect muscle for defect • Evaluate ROM of cervical spine, thoracic spine, and shoulders • Evaluate muscle strength

KEY FINDINGS	DIAGNOSTIC EVIDENCE
• The patient will likely have trigger points in the muscle that are painful • The patient will have pain with cervical motion, overhead motion, and with activity, especially after resting • Pain between shoulder blades that may extend into the neck and cause headaches	• No diagnostic evidence available

Radiating/Distal Cervical Spine Pain

Brachial Plexus Injury

HISTORY	MECHANISM OF INJURY	EVALUATION ESSENTIALS
• Patient reports having a "burner or stinger" • Acute onset • Patient reports pain, burning, numbness, or tingling from the shoulder down to the hand	• Lateral flexion with shoulder depression creating a stretching of the brachial plexus • Extension, compression, and rotation to the affected side, compressing the brachial plexus	• Upper quarter screen • Assess AROM and PROM • Brachial Plexus test stretching of the plexus • Evaluate muscle strength • Chronic "burners or stingers" need to be evaluated for the possibility of congenital spinal stenosis

KEY FINDINGS	DIAGNOSTIC EVIDENCE
• The patient will experience neuropraxia that lasts for several minutes and rarely days • Mechanism will involve either compression or a stretch at the neck, positive upper quarter screen initially that resolves quickly	• Radiographs and MRI may be indicated after multiple incidents as up to 50% of athletes with recurring injuries have been found to have spinal stenosis[13]

Radiating/Distal Cervical Spine Pain

Cervical Cord Injury

HISTORY

- Patient reports sharp pain, numbness, or tingling in a specific location or paralysis below the point of injury
- Chronic or acute onset

MECHANISM OF INJURY

- Arthritic changes causing cervical spine stenosis
- Trauma causing laceration by bony fragment, hemorrhage, cervical cord neuropraxia, or spinal shock

EVALUATION ESSENTIALS

- Palpate for sensation
- Ask patient to move toes and/or fingers
- Stabilize and activate emergency action plan

KEY FINDINGS

- The patient will have pain, weakness, and/or sensation changes below the point of injury
- Mechanism and level of cord injury determine the findings

DIAGNOSTIC EVIDENCE

- Any athlete presenting with midline neck pain or bilateral radiating symptoms in their arms or legs should be stabilized, spine boarded, and transferred to a hospital
- Radiographs, CT, and MRI may be used to determine the source of the injury[15]

Radiating/Distal Cervical Spine Pain

Cervical Spondylosis

HISTORY	MECHANISM OF INJURY	EVALUATION ESSENTIALS
• Patient reports neck pain, weakness, and decreased sensation • Chronic onset	• Abnormal wear or degeneration of the articular cartilage, and osteophytes may form • May have mineral deposits in the cervical discs	• Assess AROM and PROM • Palpate cervical spine and perform P/A glides • Evaluate muscle strength

KEY FINDINGS	DIAGNOSTIC EVIDENCE
• This will be more prevalent in patients advancing in age • There will not necessarily be a mechanism of injury, motion will be restricted, and motor function, as well as sensation, may be affected where the nerve roots are compressed	• Radiographs, CT, and MRI may be used to confirm diagnosis • There is some evidence that athletes who participated in collision sports may be more susceptible to premature cervical spondylosis[16]

Radiating/Distal Cervical Spine Pain

Intervertebral Disc Lesion/Herniation

HISTORY	MECHANISM OF INJURY	EVALUATION ESSENTIALS
• Patient reports neck pain, numbness and tingling, or radicular pain • Chronic or acute onset	• Trauma • Sustained, repetitive cervical loading during contact sports • Degenerative changes from wear and tear on the disc over time	• Assess AROM and PROM • Inspect cervical spine through palpation • Cervical compression, shoulder abduction test, and Spurling's test • Evaluate muscle strength

KEY FINDINGS	DIAGNOSTIC EVIDENCE
• The patient will have pain in the neck and decreased ROM • The patient may complain of numbness and tingling, radicular pain, and quadriparesis	• MRI may be used to confirm the diagnosis • Spurling's test (sensitivity 92%, specificity 95%)[14]

Radiating/Distal Cervical Spine Pain

Nerve Root Impingement

HISTORY	MECHANISM OF INJURY	EVALUATION ESSENTIALS
• Patient reports sharp pain and numbness or tingling in a specific location • Chronic or acute onset • Pain identified with cervical extension or rotation	• Arthritic changes • Trauma causing laceration by bony fragment, hemorrhage, cervical cord neuropraxia, or shock	• Upper quarter screen • Cervical compression, distraction, and Spurling's tests • Assess active and passive cervical spine range of motion • Evaluate muscle strength

KEY FINDINGS	DIAGNOSTIC EVIDENCE
• The patient will have pain, weakness, and sensation changes in the particular nerve root of injury • Age of the patient points more to the arthritic changes and sport usually is the acute mechanism	• MRI can determine the source of symptoms[15]

Thoracic Spine: Region/Soft Tissue Differential Diagnosis

CENTRAL

- Facet Joint Dysfunction
- Intervertebral Disc Lesion/Herniation
- Rib Dislocation/ Subluxation

PERIPHERAL

- Latissimus Dorsi Strain/Spasm
- Paraspinal Strain/ Spasm
- Rhomboid Strain/ Spasm
- Trapezius Strain/ Spasm

RADIATING/ DISTAL

- Intervertebral Disc Lesion/Herniation
- Nerve Root Impingement
- Spinal Cord Injury

Clinical Assessment of Thoracic Spine Injuries

Central Thoracic Spine Pain

Facet Joint Dysfunction

HISTORY	MECHANISM OF INJURY	EVALUATION ESSENTIALS
• Patient reports stiffness and pain • Chronic or acute onset • Pain identified with coughing, sneezing, or deep breathing	• Trauma • Poor posture • Repetitive activity leading to degenerative changes	• Standing forward flexion test and spring test • Assess prone extension, trunk lateral flexion, and trunk rotation • Evaluate mobility of facets and rib alignment

KEY FINDINGS	DIAGNOSTIC EVIDENCE
• The patient will have pain brought on by deep breathing, coughing, or sneezing that may radiate beneath the scapula • The patient likely will have history of excessive bending, arching, or twisting movement • The patient will have a facet or rib that has become hypomobile	• No diagnostic evidence available

Central Thoracic Spine Pain

Intervertebral Disc Lesion/Herniation

HISTORY	MECHANISM OF INJURY	EVALUATION ESSENTIALS
• Patient reports some kind of flexion activity and pain in his or her thoracic spine • Acute or chronic onset • Pain identified with flexion of the trunk	• Trauma • Faulty body mechanics including flexion and rotation	• Assess active and passive trunk motion • Evaluate the dermatomes of the thoracic spinal nerves • Evaluate muscle strength • Palpate for muscle guarding and or spasm

KEY FINDINGS	DIAGNOSTIC EVIDENCE
• Pain is often worse in the morning • Patient may have weakness in the abdominals and intercostals; forward bending and sitting are the most uncomfortable • Patient will ambulate slowly with slightly flexed side bend away from the side of pain	• The incidence of symptomatic thoracic disc herniation is 0.25% to 0.75% of all intervertebral disc herniations • MRI is often used to confirm diagnosis[17]

Central Thoracic Spine Pain

Rib Dislocation/Subluxation

HISTORY	MECHANISM OF INJURY	EVALUATION ESSENTIALS
• Patient reports difficulty breathing • Acute onset • Pain is severe and identified with moving	• Direct blow to the ribs • End result of a severe rib sprain	• Assess AROM and PROM and perform palpation • Visually inspect both sternum and spinal column • Evaluate ability to breathe

KEY FINDINGS	DIAGNOSTIC EVIDENCE
• Excruciating pain at the time of injury • The patient will have a visible deformity if dislocated and the bones are locked in the dislocated position • Tender over the dislocation, swelling and bruising over the rib • Pain with deep breath, cough, or laugh and possible numbness above or below dislocation	• No diagnostic evidence available

Peripheral Thoracic Spine Pain

Latissimus Dorsi Strain/Spasm

HISTORY	MECHANISM OF INJURY	EVALUATION ESSENTIALS
• Patient reports stiffness in the back • Chronic or acute onset • Pain identified with movement after resting	• Overuse and posture • Overload of the muscle, falling, or twisting	• Assess ROM of arms and shoulder • Assess pelvis for inequities such as supine to sit, ASIS and PSIS levels, and forward flexion test • Inspect muscle for defect • Evaluate muscle strength of the Latissimus dorsi

KEY FINDINGS	DIAGNOSTIC EVIDENCE
• The patient may have mid or low back pain and possibly shoulder pain • The patient will report pain with motion especially after resting • The patient may have a pelvic innominate • The patient may have pain when breathing	• No diagnostic evidence available

Peripheral Thoracic Spine Pain

Paraspinal Strain/Spasm

HISTORY	MECHANISM OF INJURY	EVALUATION ESSENTIALS
• Patient reports back pain; either unilateral or bilateral • Chronic or acute onset • Pain identified with active extension	• Sudden extension contraction on an overloaded, unprepared, or underdeveloped spine in combination with trunk rotation • Poor posture	• Assess active and passive trunk and thoracic motion • Palpate paraspinal muscles • Evaluate muscle strength

KEY FINDINGS	DIAGNOSTIC EVIDENCE
• The patient will have either local or diffuse pain • The pain will be with active extension and passive flexion • There will be no radiating or neurological symptoms	• No diagnostic evidence available

Peripheral Thoracic Spine Pain

Rhomboid Strain/Spasm

HISTORY	MECHANISM OF INJURY	EVALUATION ESSENTIALS
• Patient reports tightness or tenderness between shoulder blades • Chronic or acute onset • Pain identified with movement of the arms or with a deep breath	• Poor posture • Overload of the muscle, such as carrying too heavy of a load on one side of the body • Overuse of the muscle with rowing	• Palpate the muscle for spasm • Assess ROM of thoracic spine and shoulder motion • Inspect muscle for defect • Evaluate muscle strength

KEY FINDINGS	DIAGNOSTIC EVIDENCE
• The patient will likely have spasm within the rhomboid muscle • The patient will have pain with motion particularly overhead • The patient will experience pain with deep breathing	• No diagnostic evidence available

Peripheral Thoracic Spine Pain

Trapezius Strain/Spasm

HISTORY	MECHANISM OF INJURY	EVALUATION ESSENTIALS
• Patient reports headache and pain in upper back • Chronic or acute onset • Pain identified with motion after resting	• Carrying too heavy of a load; overloading the muscle • Poor posture • Overusing muscle • Stress	• Assess posture • Inspect muscle for defect • Evaluate ROM of cervical spine, thoracic spine, and shoulders • Evaluate muscle strength

KEY FINDINGS	DIAGNOSTIC EVIDENCE
• The patient will likely have trigger points in the muscle that are painful • The patient will have pain with overhead motion and activity, especially after resting • Pain between shoulder blades that may extend into the neck and cause headaches	• No diagnostic evidence available

Radiating/Distal Thoracic Spine Pain

Intervertebral Disc Lesion/Herniation

HISTORY	MECHANISM OF INJURY	EVALUATION ESSENTIALS
• Patient reports some kind of flexion activity and pain in his or her thoracic spine • Acute or chronic onset • Pain identified with flexion of the trunk	• Trauma • Faulty body mechanics including flexion and rotation	• Assess active and passive trunk motion • Evaluate the dermatomes, myotomes, and reflexes of the thoracic spinal nerves • Evaluate muscle strength • Palpate for muscle guarding and/or spasm

KEY FINDINGS	DIAGNOSTIC EVIDENCE
• Pain is often worse in the morning and will radiate • Patient may have weakness in the abdominals and intercostals • Forward bending and sitting are the worst • The patient will ambulate slowly with spine slightly flexed and side bend away from the side of pain	• The incidence of symptomatic thoracic disc herniation is 0.25% to 0.75% of all intervertebral disc herniations • MRI is often used to confirm diagnosis.[17]

Radiating/Distal Thoracic Spine Pain

Nerve Root Impingement

HISTORY	MECHANISM OF INJURY	EVALUATION ESSENTIALS
• Patient reports pain in a nerve distribution • Chronic or acute onset • Pain identified with specific movements	• Trauma like disc herniation • Due to stenosis	• Assess myotomes, dermatomes, and reflexes for the upper quarter • Evaluate ROM

KEY FINDINGS	DIAGNOSTIC EVIDENCE
• The patient will have radiating pain in the dermatomal pattern, weakness, sensory issues, and possible reflex changes • The patient will report numbness and or tingling • The patient will likely note pain increasing with coughing or sneezing • Pain will radiate to chest or belly.	• MRI is often used to confirm diagnosis[17]

Radiating/Distal Thoracic Spine Pain

Spinal Cord Injury

HISTORY	MECHANISM OF INJURY	EVALUATION ESSENTIALS
• Patient has history of trauma, one or both legs affected, and potentially bowel and bladder function compromised • Acute onset	• Compression of the thoracic vertebrae causing fracture • Motor vehicle accident	• Assess airway, breathing, and circulation (ABCs) • Inspect for wound • Assess for motor function • Perform dermatome and myotomes exam for the trunk, as well as the lower extremity

KEY FINDINGS	DIAGNOSTIC EVIDENCE
• The history and physical exam will be consistent with spinal cord injury • The patient will have impairment in the dermatome and myotomes at the level of injury	• CT and MRI are often used to determine the extent of bony and soft tissue injury[18]

Lumbar Spine: Region/Soft Tissue Differential Diagnosis

CENTRAL	PERIPHERAL	RADIATING/ DISTAL
• Facet Joint Dysfunction • Intervertebral Disc Lesion/Herniation • Spondylolisthesis • Spondylolysis	• Lumbar Sprain • Paraspinal Strain • Paraspinal Spasm • Sacroiliac Joint Dysfunction • Sacroiliac Joint Sprain	• Intervertebral Disc Lesion/Herniation • Nerve Root Impingement • Sciatica • Spinal Cord Injury • Spondylolisthesis

Clinical Assessment of Lumbar Spine Injuries

Central Lumbar Spine Pain

Facet Joint Dysfunction

HISTORY	MECHANISM OF INJURY	EVALUATION ESSENTIALS
• Patient reports stiffness and difficulty with standing up straight or getting up out of a chair • Chronic or acute onset • Pain identified with twisting or arching back	• Trauma • Poor posture • Repetitive activity leading to degenerative changes • Can have open or closed dysfunction	• Standing forward flexion test, spring test, and quadrant test • Assess prone extension, trunk lateral flexion, and trunk rotation • Evaluate muscle strength

KEY FINDINGS	DIAGNOSTIC EVIDENCE
• The patient will have pain and limitation in either flexion or extension with lateral flexion and rotation depending upon the dysfunction • The patient likely will have bent from the back and lifted with poor mechanics	• Quadrant test (sensitivity 100%, specificity 12% to 22%)[19]

Central Lumbar Spine Pain

Intervertebral Disc Lesion/Herniation

HISTORY

- Patient reports some kind of flexion activity and pain in his or her lower back
- Acute or chronic onset
- Pain identified with flexion of the trunk

MECHANISM OF INJURY

- Trauma
- Faulty body mechanics including flexion and rotation

EVALUATION ESSENTIALS

- Lower quarter screen
- Assess active and passive trunk motion
- Straight leg raise test, Well straight leg raise test, Milgram test, and sciatic and femoral nerve tension testing
- Evaluate muscle strength
- Palpate for muscle guarding and or spasm

KEY FINDINGS

- Pain is often worse in the morning
- Patient may have weakness in the lower limbs
- Forward bending and sitting are the worst
- The patient will ambulate slowly with slightly flexed side bend away from the side of pain
- Reflexes may be diminished.

DIAGNOSTIC EVIDENCE

- MRI (sensitivity 60% to 100%, specificity 43% to 97%)[20]
- Myotome strength testing (sensitivity 93%, specificity 27%)
- Straight leg raise test (sensitivity 92%, specificity 28%)
- Well straight leg raise test (sensitivity 28%, specificity 90%)[21]

Central Lumbar Spine Pain

Spondylolisthesis

HISTORY	MECHANISM OF INJURY	EVALUATION ESSENTIALS
• Patient reports either unilateral or bilateral pain • Chronic onset • Pain identified with extension activity	• Repetitive stress into extension	• Specific tests that are essential • Assess posture and AROM and PROM • Inspect lumbar spine for step off deformity and spasm of the para-spinals • Spring test, single leg stance test, and straight leg raise test • Evaluate muscle strength

KEY FINDINGS	DIAGNOSTIC EVIDENCE
• The patient has localized low back pain that may radiate to buttocks and posterolateral thigh, excessive lordosis, and muscular imbalances • The history and mechanism will be consistent with some repetitive extension and insidious onset of pain • Pars defect can be unilateral or bilateral; typical in adolescence and females greater than males	• Radiographs, CT scans, and MRI may all be used to confirm diagnosis[22]

Central Lumbar Spine Pain

Spondylolysis

HISTORY	MECHANISM OF INJURY	EVALUATION ESSENTIALS
• Patient reports either unilateral or bilateral pain • Chronic onset • Pain identified with extension activity	• Repetitive stress into extension	• Specific tests that are essential • Assess posture and AROM and PROM • Inspect lumbar spine for step off deformity and spasm of the para-spinals • Spring test, single leg stance test, and straight leg raise test • Evaluate muscle strength

KEY FINDINGS	DIAGNOSTIC EVIDENCE
• The patient has localized low back, excessive lordosis, and muscular imbalances • The history and mechanism will be consistent with some repetitive extension and insidious onset of pain • Pars defect can be unilateral or bilateral; typical in adolescence and females greater than males	• Radiographs, CT scans, and MRI may all be used to confirm diagnosis[22]

Peripheral Lumbar Spine Pain

Lumbar Sprain

HISTORY	MECHANISM OF INJURY	EVALUATION ESSENTIALS
• Patient reports deep sharp pain • Chronic onset • Pain identified is worse with activity	• Traumatic force overextending spine; single episode or repetitive • Can occur at any ligament in the lumbar spine with the facet joints being most common • Bend forward and twist while lifting or moving a weighted object	• Assess active and passive lumbar motion • Inspect spine for misalignments • Evaluate muscle strength

KEY FINDINGS	DIAGNOSTIC EVIDENCE
• The patient will complain of sharp, deep pain • The patient will be limited in motion by pain, and passive anteroposterior or rotational movement of the vertebrae will increase pain	• No diagnostic evidence available

Peripheral Lumbar Spine Pain

Paraspinal Strain

HISTORY	MECHANISM OF INJURY	EVALUATION ESSENTIALS
• Patient reports back pain; either unilateral or bilateral • Chronic or acute onset • Pain identified with active extension	• Sudden extension contraction on an overloaded, unprepared, or underdeveloped spine in combination with trunk rotation • Excessive lumbar lordosis	• Assess active and passive trunk and lumbar motion • Palpate paraspinal muscles • Evaluate muscle strength

KEY FINDINGS	DIAGNOSTIC EVIDENCE
• The patient will have either local or diffuse pain • The pain will be with active extension and passive flexion • There will be no radiating beyond buttocks or thigh and no neurological symptoms	• No diagnostic evidence available

Peripheral Lumbar Spine Pain

Paraspinal Spasm

HISTORY	MECHANISM OF INJURY	EVALUATION ESSENTIALS
• Patient reports tightness and spasm in the lower back • Acute onset • Pain identified with or without activity	• Reflex in response to an injury to protect the back and limit motion	• Assess active and passive trunk and lumbar motion • Palpate paraspinal muscles • Evaluate muscle strength

KEY FINDINGS	DIAGNOSTIC EVIDENCE
• The patient will have either local pain over the spasm • The pain will be with active extension and passive flexion • There will be no radiating beyond buttocks or thigh and no neurological symptoms	• No diagnostic evidence available

Peripheral Lumbar Spine Pain

Sacroiliac Joint Dysfunction

HISTORY	MECHANISM OF INJURY	EVALUATION ESSENTIALS
• Patient reports pain on one or both sides of the low back • Chronic or acute onset • Pain identified with changing positions	• Overrotating during a unilateral activity such as a golf swing • Twist with both feet planted, stumbles forward, falls backward, steps too far down landing heavy on one leg, or bends forward with knees locked during lifting	• Seated sacral flexion and extension tests, prone knee flexion test, and standing flexion test • Gillet test, sacral rocking, compression and distraction tests, and supine to sit test • Thigh thrust, Gaenslen's, sacral thrust, FABER tests • Assess ASIS and PSIS, sacral bases and ILAs, and pubic symphysis • Inspect posture and symmetry of the ischial tuberosities • Evaluate muscle strength

KEY FINDINGS	DIAGNOSTIC EVIDENCE
• This is a diagnosis by multiple positive tests • There will be palpable tenderness at the SI joint sometimes radiating down the thigh anteriorly, posteriorly, and laterally with groin pain, and testicular pain in males	• Compression test (sensitivity 63%, specificity 69%) • Distraction test (sensitivity 60%, specificity 81%) • FABER test (sensitivity 63%, specificity 76%) • Gillet test (sensitivity 43%, specificity 68%)[23]

Peripheral Lumbar Spine Pain

Sacroiliac Joint Strain

HISTORY	MECHANISM OF INJURY	EVALUATION ESSENTIALS
• Patient reports pain on one or both sides of the low back • Chronic or acute onset • Pain identified with changing positions	• Overrotating during a unilateral activity such as a golf swing • Twist with both feet planted, stumbles forward, falls backward, steps too far down landing heavy on one leg, or bends forward with knees locked during lifting	• Seated sacral flexion and extension tests and standing flexion test • Gillet test, sacral rocking, compression, and distraction tests • Assess ASIS and PSIS and sacral bases and ILAs • Inspect posture, symmetry of the ischial tuberosities • Evaluate muscle strength

KEY FINDINGS	DIAGNOSTIC EVIDENCE
• This is a diagnosis by multiple positive tests • There will be palpable tenderness at the SI joint sometimes radiating down the thigh anteriorly, posteriorly, and laterally with groin pain	• No diagnostic evidence available

Radiating/Distal Lumbar Spine Pain

Intervertebral Disc Lesion/Herniation

HISTORY	MECHANISM OF INJURY	EVALUATION ESSENTIALS
• Patient reports some kind of flexion activity and pain in his or her lower back that runs down to buttock or entire leg • Acute or chronic onset • Pain identified with flexion of the trunk	• Trauma • Faulty body mechanics including flexion and rotation resulting in overloading discs	• Lower quarter screen • Assess active and passive trunk motion • Straight leg raise test, Well straight leg raise test, Milgram test, and sciatic and femoral nerve tension testing • Evaluate muscle strength • Palpate for muscle guarding and/or spasm

KEY FINDINGS	DIAGNOSTIC EVIDENCE
• Pain is often worse in the morning • Patient may have weakness in the lower limbs; forward bending and sitting are the worst • The patient will ambulate slowly with slightly flexed side bend away from the side of pain; reflexes may be diminished	• MRI (sensitivity 60% to 100%, specificity 43% to 97%)[20] • Myotome strength testing (sensitivity 93%, specificity 27%) • Straight leg raise test (sensitivity 92%, specificity 28%) • Well straight leg raise test (sensitivity 28%, specificity 90%)[21]

Radiating/Distal Lumbar Spine Pain

Nerve Root Impingement

HISTORY	MECHANISM OF INJURY	EVALUATION ESSENTIALS
• Patient reports pain in a nerve distribution • Chronic or acute onset • Pain identified with specific movements	• Trauma-like disc herniation • Due to stenosis	• Valsalva test, straight leg raise, slump test, Milgram test, Kernig's test, Well straight leg raise test, Lasegue's test, Babinski and quadrant test • Assess myotomes and dermatomes

KEY FINDINGS	DIAGNOSTIC EVIDENCE
• The patient will have radiating pain in the dermatomal pattern, weakness, sensory issues, and possible reflex changes • The patient will report numbness and/or tingling • The quadrant test, slump test, straight leg raise tests, Valsalva, Milgram, and Kernig's tests will all be positive	• MRI (sensitivity 60% to 100%, specificity 43% to 97%)[20] • Myotome strength testing (sensitivity 93%, specificity 27%) • Straight leg raise test (sensitivity 92%, specificity 28%) • Well straight leg raise test (sensitivity 28%, specificity 90%)[21]

Radiating/Distal Lumbar Spine Pain

Sciatica

HISTORY	MECHANISM OF INJURY	EVALUATION ESSENTIALS
• Patient reports buttock pain that radiates down the posterior and medial thigh • Chronic or acute onset	• An inflammatory condition of the sciatic nerve • Compression from a disc herniation	• Straight leg raise test • Assess sciatic nerve by palpating • Be sure to rule out other pathologies

KEY FINDINGS	DIAGNOSTIC EVIDENCE
• The patient will have sharp, shooting pain down the posterior and medial thigh • Straight leg raise increases the pain • Patient with have some numbness and/or tingling along the path of the nerve • The sciatic nerve is extremely sensitive to palpation	• Straight leg raise test (sensitivity 92%, specificity 28%)[21]

Radiating/Distal Lumbar Spine Pain

Spinal Cord Injury

HISTORY	MECHANISM OF INJURY	EVALUATION ESSENTIALS
• Patient has history of trauma, one or both legs affected, and potentially bowel and bladder function compromised • Acute onset	• Diving into shallow water, gunshot wound, fall, motor vehicle accident, or industrial accident	• Ask about bowel and bladder function • Assess ABCs • Inspect for wound • Assess for motor function • Perform palpation

KEY FINDINGS	DIAGNOSTIC EVIDENCE
• The history and physical exam will be consistent with spinal cord injury • The patient will have one or both legs affected, also bowel and bladder issues along with neurological symptoms	• CT and MRI are often used to determine the extent of bony and soft tissue injury[18]

Central Lumbar Pain

Spondylolisthesis

HISTORY

- Patient reports either unilateral or bilateral pain
- Chronic onset
- Pain identified with extension activity

MECHANISM OF INJURY

- Repetitive stress into extension

EVALUATION ESSENTIALS

- Specific tests that are essential
- Assess posture and AROM and PROM
- Inspect lumbar spine for step off deformity and spasm of the para-spinals
- Spring test, single leg stance test, and straight leg raise test
- Evaluate muscle strength

KEY FINDINGS

- The patient has localized low back pain that may radiate to buttocks and posterolateral thigh, excessive lordosis, and muscular imbalances
- The history and mechanism will be consistent with some repetitive extension and insidious onset of pain
- Pars defect can be unilateral or bilateral; typical in adolescence and females greater than males

DIAGNOSTIC EVIDENCE

- Radiographs, CT scans, and MRI may all be used to confirm diagnosis[22]

Spine Pain

Injuries to Bone/Joint Surfaces

COMMON FRACTURES

- Avulsion of ligament nuchae (clay shoveler's fracture)
- Neural arch fracture
- Rib fracture (referred to spinal region)
- Spinous process fracture
- Spondylolisthesis
- Spondylolysis stress fracture
- Transverse process fracture
- Vertebral body compression fracture
- Vertebral burst fracture

Note: Stress fractures can result from mechanical loading factors and/or metabolic issues leading to insufficiency in bone health. Careful consideration must be given to patient history, activity level, and bone health.

Clinicians should also give careful consideration to acute injury mechanism and have a low tolerance for referral and radiographic evaluation following acute injury.

Paper Patient: Revisited

You should have been able to rule out several conditions secondary to knowing what structures are at the posterior lumbar spine. Your differential should have been spondylolysis versus spondylolisthesis.

Learning Activities: Practice Case

Use the blank templates provided in the Appendices to write out a differential diagnosis map and clinical findings overview for the case provided below. When working with paper patients, it is tempting to try to jump to "the answer" and come to a diagnosis. However, the visual learning approach to differential diagnosis is designed to help you consider all the possibilities for the information provided. Good luck.

Paper Patient: Low Back Pain in a Weight Lifter

History

Georgia is a 28-year-old weight lifter who complains of back pain. She was awaiting competition and hurt her back while warming up with just the bar. She reports that she bent over to pick up the bar as she has done multiple times and when she went to stand up she felt excruciating pain in her lower back. She denies radiating pain down into the buttock or the leg. The pain is sharper with certain movements, so she is not interested in moving because of the pain.

Physical Exam

Your exam reveals no tenderness to palpation over the lower back just lateral to the spinous processes of the lumbar spine levels L3 to L5. The patient has pain with passive lumbar motion for flexion and rotation. There is also pain with active motion. The patient has a negative lower quarter screen. Straight leg raise testing was negative. The patient had tightness along the paraspinals on the left greater than the right.

References

1. Deyo RA, Mirza SK, Martin BI. Back pain prevalence and visit rates: Estimates from US national surveys, 2002. *Spine*. 2006;31:2724-2727.
2. Carey TS, Evans AT, Hadler NM, et al. Acute severe low back pain: A population-based study of prevalence and care-seeking. *Spine*. 1996;21:339-344.

3. Trainor TJ, Trainor MA. Etiology of low back pain in athletes. *Curr Sports Med Rep.* 2004;3:41-46.
4. d'Hemecourt PA, Gerbino PG, Micheli LJ. Back injuries in the young athlete. *Clin Sports Med.* 2000;19:663-679.
5. Auvinen JP, Tammelin TH, Taimela SP, et al. Musculoskeletal pain in relation to different sport and exercise activities in youth. *Med Sci Sports Exerc.* 2008;40(11):1890-1900.
6. An HS, Jenis LG, Vaccaro AR. Adult spine trauma. In: Beaty JH, ed. *Orthopaedic Knowledge Update 6.* Rosemont, IL: American Academy of Orthopaedic Surgeons; 1999:653-671.
7. Watkins RG, Dillin WM. Lumbar spine injuries. In: Fu FF, Stone DA, eds. *Sports Injuries: Mechanisms, Prevention, Treatment.* Baltimore, MD: Williams & Wilkins; 1994:877-948.
8. Keene JS, Albert MJ, Springer SL, Drummond DS, Clancy WG Jr. Back injuries in college athletes. *J Spinal Disord.* 1989;2:190-195.
9. Micheli LJ, Wood R. Back pain in young athletes: Significant differences from adults in causes and patterns. *Arch Pediatr Adolesc Med.* 1995;149:15-18.
10. Bono CM. Low-back pain in athletes. *J Bone Joint Surg Am.* 2004;86-A(2):382-396.
11. Manchikanti L. Epidemiology of low back pain. *Pain Physician.* 2000;3(2):167-192.
12. Petering RC, Webb C. Treatment options for low back pain in athletes. *Sports Health.* 2011;3(6):550-555.
13. Chang D, Bosco JA. Cervical spine injuries in the athlete. *Bull NYU Hosp Jt Dis.* 2006;64(3-4):119-129.
14. Shah KC, Rajshekhar V. Reliability of diagnosis of soft cervical disc prolapse using Spurling's test. *Br J Neurosurg.* 2004;18(5):480-483.
15. Bettencourt RB, Linder MM. Treatment of neck injuries. *Prim Care.* 2013;40(2):259-269.
16. Triantafillou KM, Lauerman W, Kalantar SB. Degenerative disease of the cervical spine and its relationship to athletes. *Clin Sports Med.* 2012;31(3):509-520.
17. Baranto A, Börjesson M, Danielsson B, Hellström M, Swärd L. Acute chest pain in a top soccer player due to thoracic disc herniation. *Spine.* 2009;34(10): E359-62.
18. Looby S, Flanders A. Spine trauma. Radiol Clin North Am. 2011;49(1):129-163.
19. Cook C, Hegedus E. Diagnostic utility of clinical tests for spinal dysfunction. *Man Ther.* 2011;16(1):21-25.
20. Jarvik JG, Deyo RA. Diagnostic evaluation of low back pain with emphasis on imaging. *Ann Intern Med.* 2002;137(7):586-597.
21. van der Windt DA, Simons E, Riphagen II, et al. Physical examination for lumbar radiculopathy due to disc herniation in patients with low-back pain. *Cochrane Database Syst Rev.* 2010;17(2):CD007431.
22. McTimoney CA, Micheli LJ. Current evaluation and management of spondylolysis and spondylolisthesis. *Curr Sports Med Rep.* 2003;2(1):41-46.
23. Szadek KM, van der Wurff P, van Tulder MW, Zuurmond WW, Perez RS. Diagnostic validity of criteria for sacroiliac joint pain: A systematic review. *J Pain.* 2009;10(4):354-368.

7

The Shoulder

The glenohumeral joint of the shoulder is one important part of a greater shoulder girdle complex. The shoulder girdle includes multiple articulations, and when working properly, it allows the glenohumeral joint to enjoy 3 degrees of freedom and substantial joint range of motion. This shoulder girdle also helps bind the upper extremity portion of the appendicular skeleton to our axial skeleton. The glenohumeral joint, acromioclavicular joint, sternoclavicular joint, and the scapulothoracic articulation must work in concert to allow for full pain-free range of motion at the shoulder. Having highly mobile upper extremities has been an asset to humans as a species. However, having lots of mobility comes at a high price. Unlike the deep and stable hip, the glenohumeral joint of the shoulder exchanges stability in favor of mobility. Mobility and stability always operate on a continuum. Increasing stability means compromising mobility and vice versa. To combat this inherently unstable joint, the surrounding musculature and tendinous structures often are overworked, leading to a variety of chronic injuries (eg, musculotendinous strains, tendinosis, bursitis). This balance can create a paradox for the competitive and recreational athlete: to generate proper forces (eg, in throwers), the structures of the shoulder must have adequate laxity to achieve full range of motion and yet have the stability to inhibit subluxation. This is sometimes called the thrower's paradox.[1]

Hypermobile patients may be classified as having a multidirectional instability (MDI). This hypermobility of the shoulder is a common source of dysfunction and pain in both athletes and sedentary individuals.[2] An MDI

Winterstein AP, Clark SV. *The Athletic Trainer's Guide to Differential Diagnosis (pp 203-238).*

patient has symptomatic, abnormal glenohumeral laxity in more than one direction. Repetitive microtrauma such as that experienced by swimmers, gymnasts, volleyball players, and tennis players can lead to multidirectional instability through repetitive stretching of the shoulder capsule and ligaments. Hypermobile patients are more likely to experience overuse injury to the labrum, rotator cuff tendinosis, impingement pathologies, bursitis, and other secondary problems associated with excessive mobility.[3-6]

On the other end of the continuum are patients who develop soft tissue pathologies that are related to functional loss in motion. Patients may experience hypomobility or specific directional hypomobility of the shoulder. For instance, overhead athletes may gradually develop glenohumeral internal rotation deficits (GIRD) and associated posterior capsular tightness that present clinically as internal impingement pathologies.[7,8] The most extreme hypomobility issue for the glenohumeral joint is frozen shoulder. *Frozen shoulder syndrome,* or adhesive capsulitis, is a condition of uncertain etiology characterized by significant restriction of both active and passive shoulder motion that occurs in the absence of a known intrinsic shoulder disorder.[9] Adhesive capsulitis usually presents with a gradual onset, and patients only seek care when activities of daily living are compromised.

These examples illustrate the need for clinicians to carefully and thoughtfully evaluate patients with shoulder pain. Clinicians who understand the delicate dance between stability and mobility will be better prepared to explore the range of injuries that can present at the shoulder. The nature of sport and physical activity are such that the shoulder can be placed in compromising positions, subjected to direct blows, and required to generate and absorb great force. The sports medicine practitioner must be well versed in the possible chronic and acute injuries when discerning his or her patient's underlying problem. Once again, practitioners will be well served by creating a differential diagnosis map to aid them in their diagnostic efforts.

Paper Patient: Shoulder Pain in a Volleyball Player

History

Hannah is a 16-year-old volleyball player who complains of left side shoulder pain. She reports that she just started playing volleyball as an outside hitter and is one of the only girls who can serve overhead. She mostly has pain with just her serve during volleyball, and then when her arm is in certain positions at home. It does hurt when she carries her heavy backpack around school. She has never hurt her shoulder before. She used to be a swimmer, and she is the goalie for the soccer team. She is left-handed.

Physical Exam

Your exam reveals tenderness to palpation over the posterolateral shoulder on the left side. The patient has pain with active motion into the cock up and overhead positions. The following tests are positive: Neer's, Hawkins Kennedy, posterior impingement testing, and negative cross-over testing. The patient has pain with MMT of external rotation at 0 and 90 degrees abduction on the left, as well as with empty can testing. MMT using a break testing for 0 degrees abduction external and internal rotation, and full can testing is 5/5, 4/5 for empty can testing, and 90 degrees of abduction testing. Speed's testing is negative, as are O'Brien's and lift off testing.

The patient has laxity with a/p glide and a positive sulcus test. The patient also has 9/9 points on the Beighton Scale of hypermobility.

Clinical Decisions

Using the information from your clinical exam, ask yourself these questions to guide your clinical decision making:

- What is your differential diagnosis?
- What key findings do you see to help guide your differential?
- What are the possible injuries associated with the history and physical exam?

Start with a review of the anatomy maps and a thorough consideration of the possible injuries and conditions that are common to the shoulder. Use the differential diagnosis maps to guide your thought process and organize the possibilities. The organized synthesis of this information is the essence of clinical decision making. We will revisit this case at the end of the chapter.

Anatomy Map: Shoulder

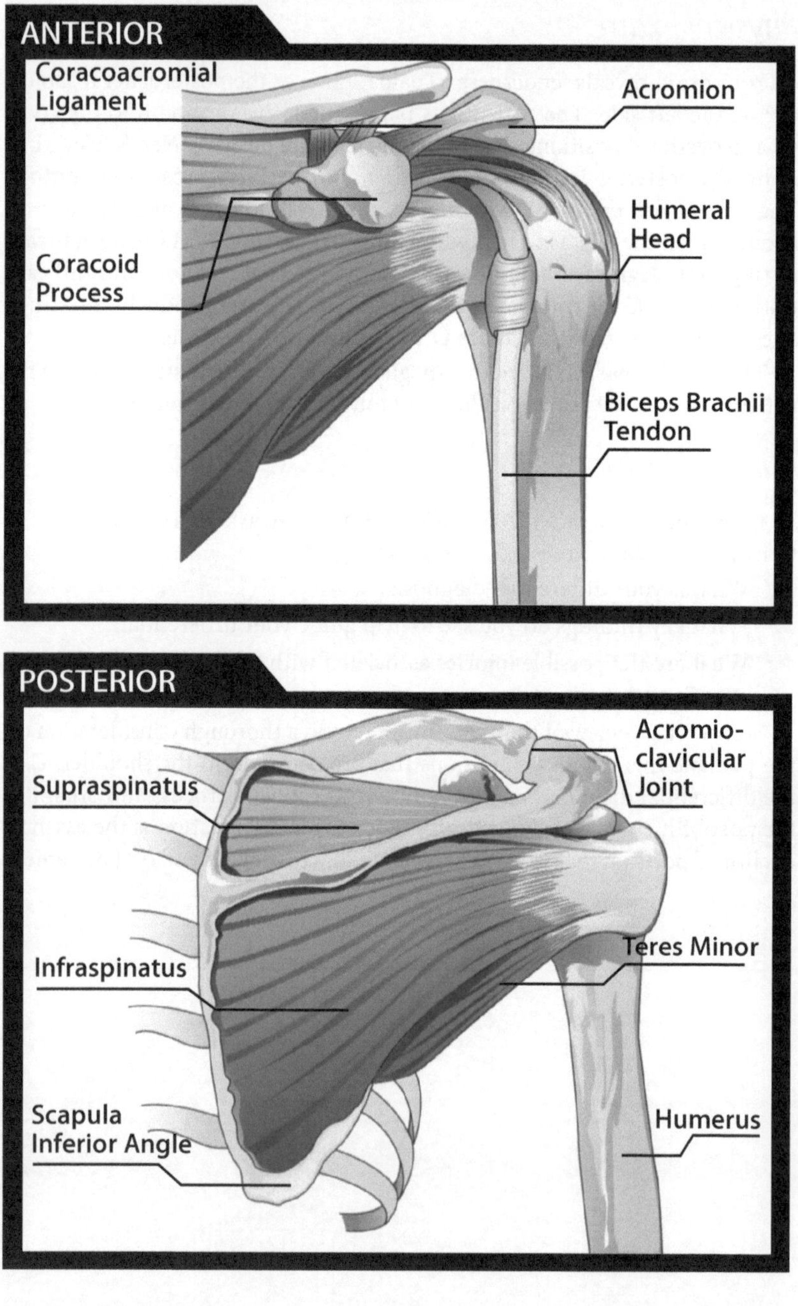

Anatomy Map: Shoulder

DEEP

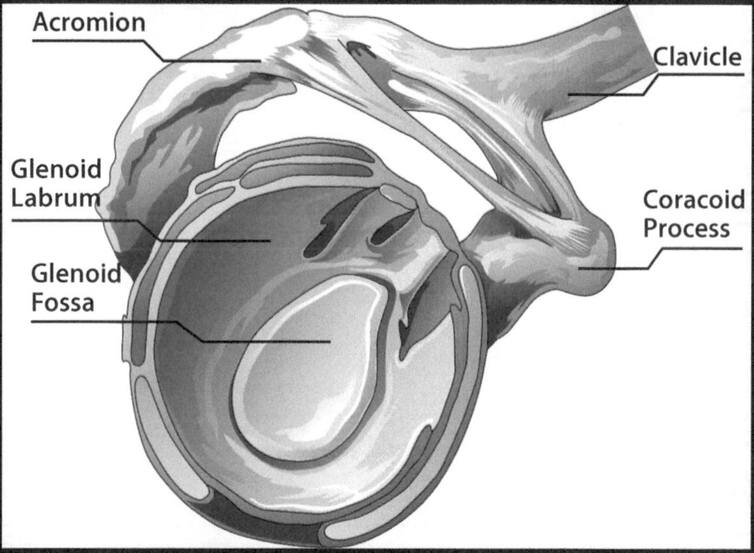

SUPERFICIAL

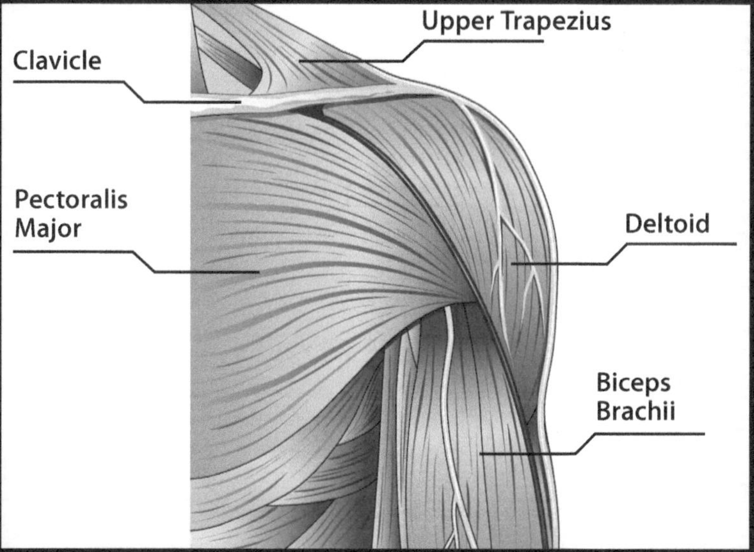

Shoulder Map: Region/Soft Tissue Differential Diagnosis

ANTERIOR

- Glenohumeral Dislocation/ Subluxation
- Chronic Anterior Instability
- Biceps Tendinopathy
- Biceps Tendon Rupture
- Pectoralis Musculotendinous Strain
- Primary Impingement Syndrome
- Secondary Impingement Syndrome
- Thoracic Outlet Syndrome (TOS)

POSTERIOR

- Labral Tear
- Posterior Glenohumeral Dislocation/ Subluxation
- Internal or Posterior Impingement Syndrome
- Posterior Glenohumeral Instability
- Scapular Dyskinesis
- Scapular Winging
- Trapezius Strain
- Trapezius Trigger Point/Spasm

MEDIAL

- Scalene Muscle Strain
- Sternoclavicular (SC) Sprain
- Sternocleido-mastoid Strain

LATERAL

- Acromioclavicular Joint Sprain
- Glenohumeral Adhesive Capsulitis
- Deltoid Muscle Strain
- Parsonage Turner Syndrome
- Rotator Cuff Strain
- Rotator Cuff Tendinopathy
- Subacromial Bursitis

Shoulder Girdle

Injuries to Bone/Joint Surfaces

COMMON FRACTURES

- **Clavicle**—Neer Classification of clavicle fractures
  - Proximal third (least common)
    - Type I—Minimal displacement
    - Type II—Significant displacement
    - Type III—Articular surface fracture
    - Type IV—Epiphyseal separation
    - Type V—Comminuted
  - Middle third (most common (80%); identified by degree of displacement)
  - Distal third (most complex of clavicle fractures)
    - Type I—Minimal displacement
    - Type II—Fracture medial to coracoclavicular ligaments
    - Type III—Articular surface fracture
    - Type IV—Ligaments intact to periosteum with displacement of proximal fragment
    - Type V—Comminuted
- **Scapula**
  - Uncommon; only 3% to 5% of all shoulder fractures
  - Described by anatomic location. The scapula may be divided into five areas: glenoid neck, intra-articular glenoid, scapula body and spine, coracoid, and acromion.
- **Proximal Humerus Fractures** (Most common in elderly)
  - Complex classification based on angulation, displacement, and intra versus extra articular
  - Compression fractures to humeral head common post gleno–humeral dislocation
  - Epiphyseal injuries must be considered in adolescents

Clinical Assessment of Shoulder Injuries

Anterior Shoulder Pain

Glenohumeral Dislocation/Subluxation

HISTORY	MECHANISM OF INJURY	EVALUATION ESSENTIALS
• Patient may report an acute injury or discomfort associated with chronic instability • Pain in anterior and inferior region of the shoulder • Patient with subluxing GH joint may describe a sensation of instability with abduction/external rotation	• Acute MOI • Fall on an outstretched arm • Chronic instability may become symptomatic with specific motions	• Observe the contour of the deltoid for deformity • Assess motion and strength if possible • Perform apprehension/relocation testing • Sulcus sign or inferior glide • Upper quarter screen

KEY FINDINGS	DIAGNOSTIC EVIDENCE
• With a history of trauma must determine is GH joint is in place • Pain, flattened deltoid, and patient supporting arm are indications the GH joint is dislocated and not reduced • Reduction and proper referral is warranted • Patient with recurrent subluxation may describe a "sliding" sensation	• All first time dislocations should be referred for a radiographic evaluation • Apprehension (sensitivity 65.6%, specificity 95.4%) • Relocation (sensitivity 64.6%, specificity 90.2%)[10]

Anterior Shoulder Pain

Chronic Anterior Instability

HISTORY	MECHANISM OF INJURY	EVALUATION ESSENTIALS
• Patient may report discomfort associated with chronic instability • Pain in anterior and inferior region of the shoulder • Sensation of instability with abduction/external rotation (90/90) • DIfficulty with functional activities	• Generalized laxity (genetic) • Previous acute GH joint dislocation • Chronic instability may become symptomatic with specific motions	• Assess motion and strength • Perform apprehension/relocation testing • Sulcus sign or inferior glide • Upper quarter screen • Assess GH joint for labral damage (O'Brien, jerk, and grind tests) • Functional assessment

KEY FINDINGS	DIAGNOSTIC EVIDENCE
• Patient with recurrent subluxation may describe a "sliding" sensation • Correlation of physical exam to logical history is essential	• Ultrasound (sensitivity 20% to 100%, specificity 25% to 90%) • MRA (sensitivity 80% to 100%, specificity 50% to 100%)[11]

Anterior Shoulder Pain

Biceps Tendinopathy

HISTORY	MECHANISM OF INJURY	EVALUATION ESSENTIALS
• Patient may report tenderness over the anterior upper arm at biceps tendon • Pain with overhead and throwing motions • May report snapping in the front of the shoulder	• Chronic MOI • Repetitive overhead activities • Biceps tendinopathy is often a secondary issue to other GH conditions	• Observe the contour and tone of biceps for deformity • Assess motion and strength (MMT) of GH joint and biceps • Palpate for pain • Special tests for biceps tendon (Speed's, Yergason's, and biceps load testing)

KEY FINDINGS	DIAGNOSTIC EVIDENCE
• Patients are classically tender over the long head of the biceps in the bicipital groove • Pain worsens with overhead lifting or activity • Night pain is common • Since biceps tendinopathy is often a secondary condition it is imperative that clinicians determine underlying cause of stress on biceps tendon.	• Speed's test (sensitivity 49% to 71%, specificity 60% to 85%) • Yergason's test (sensitivity 14% to 75%, specificity 78% to 81%) • Biceps palpation (sensitivity 57%, specificity 74%)[10]

Anterior Shoulder Pain

Biceps Tendon Rupture

HISTORY	MECHANISM OF INJURY	EVALUATION ESSENTIALS
• Patient may report an acute injury • Sudden and intense pain • Patient may report an audible pop • Trauma, sport participation, or heaving weightlifing may be described in the history	• Acute MOI • Fall on an outstretched arm • Chronic instability may become symptomatic with specific motions	• Observe the shape of the biceps for deformity • Assess motion and strength if possible • Palpate muscle and tendon structures • Ludington test to observe deformity

KEY FINDINGS	DIAGNOSTIC EVIDENCE
• Popeye deformity in upper arm, audible pop or snap reported by patient, ecchymosis seen initially • Typically an injury seen in middle aged patients with history of tendinopathy • Younger individuals may rupture the biceps tendon following a traumatic fall, during heavy weightlifting, or during sporting activities	• Proximal ruptures are the most common (90% to 97%) with involvement of the long head of the biceps • Normally diagnosed through history and physical exam; ultrasonography of the anterior shoulder can provide a useful and reliable evaluation of the tissue integrity and aid in treatment planning[12]

Anterior Shoulder Pain

Pectoralis Musculotendinous Strain

HISTORY	MECHANISM OF INJURY	EVALUATION ESSENTIALS
• Patient may report acute episode of painful injury • May describe pain at muscle origin (along sternum), mid belly of the muscle, or muscle insertion (at humerus) • Pain with lifting heavy objects	• Acute MOI • Associated with lifting too heavy of an object • Overstretch of muscle tissues in horizontal abduction	• Assess AROM of the GH joint for actions of the pectoralis (humeral flexion, adduction, and medial humeral rotation) • Observe and palpate for tissue deformity • Manual muscle testing for pectoralis major and minor

KEY FINDINGS	DIAGNOSTIC EVIDENCE
• Injury consistent with mechanism • Common injury with weight lifters • Implicated as a common injury secondary to anabolic steriod abuse	• ~47% of cases occur during bench press • MRI may be used to confirm diagnosis[13]

Anterior Shoulder Pain

Primary Impingement Syndrome

HISTORY	MECHANISM OF INJURY	EVALUATION ESSENTIALS
• Patient will report anterior or anterolateral shoulder pain • Painful arc of motion moving arm overhead starting at about 60 degrees • May report night pain • Pain with overhead activities in general	• Chronic MOI • Repetitive overuse mechanism • Poor posture and poor scapular mechanics are contributing factors • Anatomical variations of acromion also contribute to primary impingement	• Assess motion and strength (MMT) of GH joint (rotator cuff) • Palpate distal rotator cuff tendons • Evaluate scapular mechanics and postural positioning • Special tests (crossover, Neer's, Hawkins Kennedy, empty can)

KEY FINDINGS	DIAGNOSTIC EVIDENCE
• Patients over 30 years old who present with impingement signs and symptoms may be hypomobile • Knowledge of anatomical variations of the the acromion (eg, hooked acromion type 2+) may be useful for treatment planning	• Neer's test (sensitivity 72%, specificity 60%) • Hawkins Kennedy test (sensitivity 80%, specificity 56%)[10]

Anterior Shoulder Pain

Secondary Impingement Syndrome

HISTORY	MECHANISM OF INJURY	EVALUATION ESSENTIALS
• Patient will report anterior or anterolateral shoulder pain • Painful arc of motion moving arm overhead starting at about 60 degrees • Aching pain • Pain with overhead activities in general	• Chronic MOI • Repetitive overuse mechanism • Poor posture, poor scapular mechanics, and glenohumeral instability are contributing factors	• Assess motion and strength (MMT) of GH joint (rotator cuff) • Palpate distal rotator cuff tendons • Evaluate scapular mechanics, posture, and glenohumeral stability • Special tests (Crossover, Neer's, Hawkins Kennedy, Empty Can)

KEY FINDINGS	DIAGNOSTIC EVIDENCE
• Secondary impingement is secondary to other GH issues • Patients under 30 years old who present with impingement symptoms may be hypermobile • Cannot control motion due to instability, poor RC strength, and scapular dyskinesis • Determination of underlying causes is critical	• Neer's test (sensitivity 72%, specificity 60%) • Hawkins Kennedy test (sensitivity 80%, specificity 56%) • Painful arc (sensitivity 53%, specificity 76%)[10]

Anterior Shoulder Pain

Thoracic Outlet Syndrome

HISTORY	MECHANISM OF INJURY	EVALUATION ESSENTIALS
• Patient may report neurologic symptoms, vascular symptoms, or both • Often describes pain and numbness • Discoloration of skin may be seen in extreme cases • Numbness and tingling with overhead activity	• Chronic MOI • Repetitive motions secondary to tightness of the scalene muscles, pectoralis minor muscles or first rib compression on the neurovascular bundle	• Comprehensive evaluation of the GH joint and cervical spine are key to differential • Assess motion, strength, and movement patterns • Specials tests: Roos, Allen's, Adson, Military brace test

KEY FINDINGS	DIAGNOSTIC EVIDENCE
• Sometimes described as neurogenic TOS or vascular TOS depending on structures being compressed • Evaluaton of activity mechanics and postural positions is essential • Often a diagnosis of exclusion with false positives of special tests fairly common • Cervical spine is key differential for any upper extremity neurologic symptoms	• Adson test (sensitivity 79%, specificity 76%) • Roos test (sensitivity 84%, specificity 30%)[14]

Posterior Shoulder Pain

Labral Tear

HISTORY	MECHANISM OF INJURY	EVALUATION ESSENTIALS
• Patient describes pain in the posterior aspect of the shoulder with activity • May report night pain, aching pain, or a feeling of instability • Describes sensation of clicking or catching with specific movements.	• Acute MOI • Fall on an outstretched hand (FOOSH), blocking opponent with arms out stretched, or other trauma • Chronic onset can occur with repetitive activities and associated instabilities	• Full evaluation of the GH joint is needed • Assess active and passive motion • MMT • Assess GH joint stability • Special tests for labrum (O'Brien's, crank, and clunk test)

KEY FINDINGS	DIAGNOSTIC EVIDENCE
• Sensations of popping or clicking posteriorly with activity is a common indicator of labral pathology • Commonly associated with GH dislocation	• O'Brien's test (sensitivity 53% to 91%, specificity 40% to 92%) • Crank test (sensitivity 57.3%, specificity 72.6%)[10] • MRI (sensitivity 76%, specificity 87%) • MRA (sensitivity 88%, specificity 93%)[15]

Posterior Shoulder Pain

Posterior Glenohumeral Dislocation/Subluxation

HISTORY	MECHANISM OF INJURY	EVALUATION ESSENTIALS
• Patient may report an acute injury such as a direct blow or other trauma • Pain at the posterior shoulder • Describes loss of function at GH joint	• Acute MOI • Forceful contraction of internal rotator or direct blow to anterior GH joint with a forward flexed arm	• Observe the contour of the deltoid for deformity • Assess motion and strength if possible • Palpation for proper GH joint position • Radiographs can confirm dislocation with the definitive test in an axillary view

KEY FINDINGS	DIAGNOSTIC EVIDENCE
• Glenohumeral dislocations are less common and not as obvious in the posterior direction; this can be a missed diagnosis	• Posterior shoulder dislocation accounts for ~2% to 5% of all dislocations • 60% to 79% are missed on initial evaluation • 65% had associated injuries • Radiographs, CT, and MRI may all be used to confirm diagnosis and evaluate surrounding structures[16]

Posterior Shoulder Pain

Internal or Posterior Impingement Syndrome

HISTORY	MECHANISM OF INJURY	EVALUATION ESSENTIALS
• Patient reports posterior shoulder pain • Pain moving arm overhead starting at about 90 degrees • Describes limits in internal rotation and possible pain with IR	• Chronic onset MOI • Contributing factors include overuse, poor scapular mechanics, glenohumeral instability, and GIRD	• Identify location of pain • Full evaluation of GH joint including motion, strength (MMT), and joint stability • Special test (posterior impingement test [in 90/90 apprehension position apply anterior humeral translation])

KEY FINDINGS	DIAGNOSTIC EVIDENCE
• Common injury among repetitive overhead athletes, patients with excessive external rotation, and those with GIRD	• Posterior impingement test (sensitivity 75.5%, specificity 85%)[17]

Posterior Shoulder Pain

Posterior Glenohumeral Instability

HISTORY	MECHANISM OF INJURY	EVALUATION ESSENTIALS
• Patient will present with a sensation of posterior instability of glenohumeral joint; describes shoulder as "sliding out the back" • May describe activities with extended arms and longitudinal force to GH joint (eg, pass blocking in football)	• Acute MOI or chronic onset (repetitive forces) • Chronic instability may become symptomatic with specific motions	• Assess motion and strength if possible • Perform posterior apprehension test • Joint play assessment (posterior glide) posterior glide • MRI to assess integrity of the coracohumeral and superior glenohumeral ligament may be needed

KEY FINDINGS	DIAGNOSTIC EVIDENCE
• Patients with posterior instability may have more global multidirectional instability—it is essential to assess all directions • Instability may be accompanied by a labral injury • Diagnostic imaging may reveal genetic anomalies to the glenoid or humeral head	• Posterior instability accounts for only 2% to 10% of unstable shoulders • MRA is 90% to 94% accurate in the evaluation of posterior instability and labral pathology[18]

Posterior Shoulder Pain

Scapular Dyskinesis

HISTORY	MECHANISM OF INJURY	EVALUATION ESSENTIALS
• Patient reports shoulder pain • Most likely will report a gradual onset of shoulder pain • May participate in an activity with repetitive overhead shoulder motion	• Scapular dyskinesis is usually associated with poor posture or secondary to trauma • Most often found as part of an evaluation for other problems (eg, impingement syndrome, rotator cuff strain injury)	• Inspect patient posture • Full glenohumeral joint assessment • AROM and PROM • Scapular kinematics (assess scapulohumeral rhythm) • Measurement of medial scapular border in relation to spine for bilataral comparison

KEY FINDINGS	DIAGNOSTIC EVIDENCE
• Essential to determine impact of scapular dyskinesis on overall glenohumeral joint function • Scapular dyskinesis is usually a secondary finding with patients presenting for other shoulder pain issues • Keen observation skills and practice is required to note subtle deviations in normal scapluar control	• A 1.5-cm difference from side to side when measuring distance from medial border to spine is considered abnormal[19]

Posterior Shoulder Pain

Scapular Winging

HISTORY	MECHANISM OF INJURY	EVALUATION ESSENTIALS
• Patient reports abnormal position of scapula, usually unilateral • May be painful • Can affect lifting, pushing, or pulling of light or heavy objects	• Acute: trauma (eg, direct blow or twisting of neck and shoulders causing damage to the long thoracic nerve which innervates the serratus anterior muscle) • Chronic usually repetitive in nature • Cause can be non-mechanical (eg, viral illness, drug reaction)	• Inspect patient posture and musculature • Full glenohumeral assessment • AROM and PROM not movement into abduction to assess scapulohumeral rhythm and position of the scapula • MMT serratus anterior

KEY FINDINGS	DIAGNOSTIC EVIDENCE
• Full neuruological assessment of associated nerve function may be necessary • Essential to determine impact of scapular winging on overall glenohumeral joint function • Scapular winging may be a secondary finding with patients presenting for other shoulder pain issues.	• No diagnostic evidence available

Posterior Shoulder Pain

Trapezius Strain

HISTORY

- Patient reports posterior shoulder pain about the scapula possibly into their neck
- May describe either an acute injury incident or a more chronic onset
- Posterior shoulder pain identified with lifting a heavy object or carrying heavy objects

MECHANISM OF INJURY

- Acute MOI or chronic onset
- Acute: lifting a heavy object
- Chronic: carrying heavy bag or pack on one side of the body
- Chronic onset is also associated with poor posture (rounded shoulders and head forward); prolonged slumped, seated position

EVALUATION ESSENTIALS

- Assess manual muscle test for all fiber configurations of the trapezius (upper, middle, and lower fibers)
- Inspect patient posture and musculature

KEY FINDINGS

- Evaluation of GH joint and cervical spine necessary to rule out other sources of pain
- Common injury among weight lifters, people who have recently traveled and lifted heavy baggage, or occupations that require carry items over the shoulder (eg, postal carrier)

DIAGNOSTIC EVIDENCE

- No diagnostic evidence available

Posterior Shoulder Pain

Trapezius Trigger Points/Spasm

HISTORY	MECHANISM OF INJURY	EVALUATION ESSENTIALS
• Patient may report stiff neck, mid back pain, pain about the scapula, or an aching in the shoulder • May describe acute onset with heavy lifting or chronic onset. • Pain identified with activities of daily living involving lifting or carrying objects.	• Acute: lifting a heavy object • Chronic: carrying objects, repetitive shoulder motions (eg, kayaking), or a unilateral repetitive overhead sport • Chronic onset is also associated with poor posture and muscle imbalances • Slumped seated postion.	• Assess manual muscle test for all fiber configurations of the trapezius (upper, middle, and lower fibers) • Inspect patient posture in standing position and inspect musculature • Palpate for trigger points throughout entire trapezius muscle

KEY FINDINGS	DIAGNOSTIC EVIDENCE
• You will be able to palpate the trigger point and it will reproduce the patient's pain in the referral pattern for the trapezius	• Prevalence of ~20% in the general population[20]

Medial Shoulder Pain

Scalene Muscle Strain

HISTORY	MECHANISM OF INJURY	EVALUATION ESSENTIALS
• Patient reports possible anterior, lateral, or posterior neck pain • May describe deep aching pain (like a tooth ache); sometimes at night • Patient may have numbness and tingling down the arm • May be worse at night	• Acute MOI may involve a whiplash-style sports injury • Long-term tightness of the scalenes may be secondary to poor postural positions	• Palpation of the scalenes and their origins and insertions • AROM and PROM testing • MMT (lateral neck flexion) • Evaluate inspiration (elevation of rib cage)

KEY FINDINGS	DIAGNOSTIC EVIDENCE
• Muscle spasm and persistent tension in the scalene muscle group is contributor to chronic neck pain • Scalenes can be one contributor to thoracic outlet syndrome (TOS) • Clavicular depression may be observed	• No diagnostic evidence available

Medial Shoulder Pain

Sternoclavicular Joint Injury

HISTORY	MECHANISM OF INJURY	EVALUATION ESSENTIALS
• Patient reports pain at the promixal clavicle (SC joint) possibly into his or her neck • May describe instability of the joint depending upon severity of the sprain • May report pain in SC with GH motions (overhead and horizontal adduction)	• Acute MOI is most common • Traumatic injury (eg, car accident or sports injury) • Common sports MOI: landing on point of the shoulder, FOOSH, or direct blow	• Palpation of the SC joint • ROM testing for GH joint and shoulder girdle • Joint stability assessment by moving proximal clavicle • Radiographs

KEY FINDINGS	DIAGNOSTIC EVIDENCE
• The SC joint can be dislocated • Even a stable joint may have painful clicking, grating, or popping with a ligamentous or capsular injury • Proximal clavicle often is one of the last epiphyseal plates to close well into young adulthood; this must be considered in patients slow to respond to treatment	• Computed tomography is often used to assess the integrity of the SC joint • MRI may be used to evaluate the intra-articular disc and surrounding soft tissue structures[21]

Medial Shoulder Pain

Sternocleidomastoid Strain

HISTORY	MECHANISM OF INJURY	EVALUATION ESSENTIALS
• Patient reports whiplash injury • Pain can be in the muscle at the site of injury or referred to posterior and lateral neck • Patient may complain of a headache	• Acute MOI is most common • Traumatic injury (eg, car accident or sports injury) • Whiplash-style MOI	• Palpation of the SCM and its origin and insertions • AROM and PROM testing • MMT (flexion, lateral neck flexion, and rotation)

KEY FINDINGS	DIAGNOSTIC EVIDENCE
• Muscle spasm and persistent tension in the sternocleidomastoid muscle is a contributor to chronic neck pain • Ecchymosis and edema may be present in severe cases	• No diagnostic evidence available

Lateral Shoulder Pain

Acromioclavicular Joint Sprain

HISTORY

- Patient reports history of acute injury
- Describes a fall on a tucked or outstretched arm
- Reports pain with motion particularly horizontal adduction

MECHANISM OF INJURY

- Acute MOI
- Direct blow to point of the shoulder
- FOOSH

EVALUATION ESSENTIALS

- Observe for AC deformity
- Assess motion and strength
- Special tests (spring test [piano key sign], AC joint compression testing)
- Palpation of related bony structures
- Functional assessment

KEY FINDINGS

- May present with a range of mild to significant deformity; classification up to 6 degrees of severity (Rockwood classification)
- Logical history consistent with clinical findings
- Pain with horizontal adduction (crossover) is classic indicator

DIAGNOSTIC EVIDENCE

- Horizontal adduction test (sensitivity 77%)
- Rockwood Classification
  - Type 1: AC sprain
  - Type 2: AC ligament torn
  - Type 3: AC and CC ligaments torn
  - Type 4: Posterior clavicle dislocation
  - Type 5: Ligaments, deltoid/trap torn
  - Type 6: Inferior clavicle dislocation[22]

Lateral Shoulder Pain

Glenohumeral Adhesive Capsulitis

HISTORY	MECHANISM OF INJURY	EVALUATION ESSENTIALS
• Patient reports intense pain in the shoulder at all times • Presents with a lack of motion • Typically an older patient • Patients who are post surgical, diabetic, or peri-menopausal women are at increased risk	• Idiopathic • Characterized by contracted and thickened joint capsule with little synovial fluid	• Evaluation will reveal passive and active restriction in joint play assessment • Lack of active and passive motions • History is key to diagnosis and essential to evaluation

KEY FINDINGS	DIAGNOSTIC EVIDENCE
• Patients with excessive pain • Classic pattern of motion loss with loss of abduction and external rotation • Loss of motion and pain will differ in phases of capsulitis • Typically middle aged female patient with loss of motion in non-dominant arm • More common in those with metabolic issues (eg, diabetes)	• Estimated to affect 2% of the general population • Generally occurs in people between 40 to 60 years old • Diabetics have a 10% to 20% lifetime risk of developing adhesive capsulitis[23]

Lateral Shoulder Pain

Deltoid Muscle Strain

HISTORY	MECHANISM OF INJURY	EVALUATION ESSENTIALS
• Patient complains of excruciating pain • Capsular pattern of motion loss (abduction and external rotation) • Pain identified with forward flexion, abduction, or extension of the shoulder	• Acute or chronic MOI • Direct trauma or blow to the shoulder • Overuse of the muscle without adequate rest • Forced eccentric contraction of the shoulder	• Assess AROM of the GH joint for actions of the deltoid (GH flexion, abduction, and extension) • Observe and palpate tissue for deformity • MMT for all 3 portions of the deltoid

KEY FINDINGS	DIAGNOSTIC EVIDENCE
• This could be placed in either the anterior, posterior, or lateral portion of the map as the muscle has 3 portions • Presence of rotator cuff injury may cause deltoid to compensate in GH flexion, elevation, and abduction • Common site of referred pain for other shoulder pathologies (eg, rotator cuff injury, labral injury, biceps tendon, AC joint injury, shoulder dislocation, humeral fracture, or soft tissue contusion)	• No diagnostic evidence available

Lateral Shoulder Pain

Parsonage Turner Syndrome

HISTORY	MECHANISM OF INJURY	EVALUATION ESSENTIALS
• Patients may report a sudden onset of severe pain across shoulder and upper arm • Symptoms sometimes radiate down arm • Depending upon the stage patient may note weakness and not pain	• Idiopathic condition • May present after injury, viral infection, or immunization	• Parsonage Turner syndrome is often a diagnosis of exclusion • MRI to assess nerves and soft tissue is key • Association of history to findings may point toward diagnosis • MMT for specific weakness • Evaluation of pain patterns

KEY FINDINGS	DIAGNOSTIC EVIDENCE
• If assessment of the shoulder does not lead to clear diagnosis, Parsonage Turner syndrome must be ruled out • Sometimes called acute brachial neuropathy and acute brachial radiculitis • Differential diagnosis is essential; differentiate from cervical radiculopathy • Seen most often in young to middle aged adult males	• Incidence of 1.64 cases per 100,000 people • 25% precededed by viral illness • EMG is often used to assess muscle innervation • MRI is often indicated to assess the inflammatory responses in nerves[24]

Lateral Shoulder Pain

Rotator Cuff Strain

HISTORY

- Patient reports pain in the shoulder often runs down the lateral arm
- Most patients report either a fall or lifting or pulling injury
- Pain identified with reaching overhead, behind the back, pulling or lifting things, and sleeping on the injured side

MECHANISM OF INJURY

- May be acute or chronic onset injury
- FOOSH
- Repetitive overhead activity
- Lifting or pulling something heavy
- Chronic onset is related to posture or repetitive stress

EVALUATION ESSENTIALS

- Specific tests for the rotator cuff: full can (scaption), empty can, drop arm test, lift off test
- Assess patient for atrophy or deformity
- Inspect posture
- Evaluate muscle strength of each individual rotator cuff muscle

KEY FINDINGS

- This may be more of a wear and tear depending upon age of patient >40 years
- Significant strain injury resulting in loss of motion and GH function should be referred
- The referral pattern of pain for the rotator cuff is down the lateral arm sometimes right at deltoid insertion

DIAGNOSTIC EVIDENCE

- Empty can test (sensitivity 53% to 89%, specificity 54% to 82%)
- Full can test (sensitivity 86%, specificity 57%)
- Drop arm test (sensitivity 10% to 35%, specificity 88% to 98%)
- Lift off test (sensitivity 17% to 62%, specificity 60% to 98%)[25]

Lateral Shoulder Pain

Rotator Cuff Tendinopathy

HISTORY	MECHANISM OF INJURY	EVALUATION ESSENTIALS
• Patient reports anterior/lateral shoulder pain • May describe pain moving arm overhead (>60 degrees abduction) • Night pain • Pain going down the arm to the deltoid • May have popping or cracking sounds	• Chronic MOI • Repetitive overuse mechanism • Poor posture and poor scapular mechanics are contributing factors • Anatomical variations of acromion also contribute to rotator cuff tendinopathy	• Assess motion and strength (MMT) of GH joint (rotator cuff) • Palpate distal rotator cuff tendons • Evaluate scapular mechanics and postural positioning • Special tests (full can [scaption and Gerber lift off test])

KEY FINDINGS	DIAGNOSTIC EVIDENCE
• Patient will have pain at rest as tendinopathy progresses • Rotation cuff weakness • GH instability • History of injury to shoulder specifically the glenohumeral joint • Knowledge of anatomical variations of the the acromion (eg, hooked acromion type 2+) may be useful for treatment planning	• Empty can test (sensitivity 53% to 89%, specificity 54% to 82%) • Full can test (sensitivity 86%, specificity 57%) • Lift off test (sensitivity 17% to 62%, specificity 60% to 98%)[25]

Lateral Shoulder Pain

Subacromial Bursitis

HISTORY

- Patient describes localized subacromial space pain
- Painful arc of motion moving arm overhead
- Pain with overhead activities in general

MECHANISM OF INJURY

- Chronic onset overuse injury
- Poor posture and poor scapular mechanics are contributing factors in chronic onset cases
- Bursa may be inflammed secondary to trauma

EVALUATION ESSENTIALS

- Assess motion and strength (MMT) of GH joint (rotator cuff)
- Palpate structures in subacromial space
- Evaluate scapular mechanics and posture
- Special tests (Neer's, Hawkins Kennedy, and crossover)

KEY FINDINGS

- Location of pain under the acromion with shoulder testing is a key finding
- Patients will display a classic painful arc pattern with overhead activity
- Bursal inflammation often produces a "crunchy" sound or sensation (crepitus)

DIAGNOSTIC EVIDENCE

- Neer's test (sensitivity 72%, specificity 60%)
- Hawkins Kennedy test (sensitivity 80%, specificity 56%)[10]

Paper Patient: Revisited

You should have been able to rule out several conditions secondary to knowing what structures are at the posterior and lateral shoulder. Your differential should have been posterior impingement versus subacromial impingement secondary to multidirectional instability.

Learning Activities: Practice Case

Use the blank templates provided in the Appendices to write out a differential diagnosis map and clinical findings overview for the case provided below. When working with paper patients, it is tempting to try to jump to "the answer" and come to a diagnosis. However, the visual learning approach to differential diagnosis is designed to help you consider all the possibilities for the information provided. Good luck.

Paper Patient: Bilateral Shoulder Symptoms in a College Student

History

Anna is a 24-year-old vet school student who comes to clinic complaining of bilateral shoulder pain and numbness and tingling into her arms and hands. She notices this most in her lab classes because she has dropped instruments when trying to do a dissection. She has a long history of hypermobility, having had knee issues when she was in high school. She reports that she has no stamina in her arms to hold them out at a 90-degree angle in front of her. She can move them out to the side, but not without symptoms. She reports that the right side (her dominant side) is more debilitating because it affects everything she does with her right arm. She denies any neck pain or previous injury to her neck or shoulders.

Physical Exam

The patient has all 9 points on the Beighton Scale of hypermobility. She has no focal tenderness to palpation. She has a weak grip bilaterally. Her upper extremity strength was 4/5 for internal and external rotation at 0 degrees abduction; this caused her pain. Abduction to 90 degrees is 3/5 with symptoms of numbness and tingling. Allen's and Adson's tests are positive. The patient has symptoms with Roos test starting within 10 seconds. The patient has pain with Neer's, Hawkins Kennedy, and cross-over testing, and she also notes numbness and tingling starting at 90 degrees of motion.

Testing of her dermatome patterns reveals a difference between the left and right, but she felt that both sides were not as sensitive to the touch. Her reflexes are within normal limits for the upper extremity. Her myotomes for the upper quarter screen are diminished, with the right being weaker than the left.

References

1. Wilk KE, Meister K, Andrews JR. Current concepts in the rehabilitation of the overhead throwing athlete. *Am J Sports Med.* 2002;30:136-151.
2. Levine WN, Prickett WD, Prymka M, Yamaguchi K. Treatment of the athlete with multidirectional shoulder instability. *Orthop Clin North Am.* 2001;32(3): 475-484.
3. Cowderoy GA, Lisle DA, O'Connell PT. Overuse and impingement syndromes of the shoulder in the athlete. *Magn Reson Imaging Clin North Am.* 2009;17(4): 577-593.
4. Cassas KJ, Cassettari-Wayhs A. Childhood and adolescent sports-related overuse injuries. *Am Fam Physician.* 2006;73(6):1014-1022.
5. Reinold MM, Gill TJ. Current concepts in the evaluation and treatment of the shoulder in overhead-throwing athletes, part 1: Physical characteristics and clinical examination. *Sports Health.* 2010;2(1): 39-50.
6. Wolf JM, Cameron KL, Owens BD. Impact of joint laxity and hypermobility on the musculoskeletal system. *J Am Acad Orthop Surg.* 2011;19(8):463-471.
7. Tyler TF, Nicholas SJ, Lee SJ, Mullaney M, McHugh MP. Correction of posterior shoulder tightness is associated with symptom resolution in patients with internal impingement. *Am J Sports Med.* 2010;38(1): 114-119.
8. Myers JB, Laudner KG, Pasquale MR, Bradley JP, Lephart SM. Glenohumeral range of motion deficits and posterior shoulder tightness in throwers with pathologic internal impingement. *Am J Sports Med.* 2006;34(3):385-391.
9. Zuckerman JD, Cuomo F, Rokito S. Definition and classification of frozen shoulder: A consensus approach. *J Shoulder Elbow Surg.* 1994;3(1): S72.
10. Hegedus EJ, Goode AP, Cook CE, et al. Which physical examination tests provide clinicians with the most value when examining the shoulder? Update of a systematic review with meta-analysis of individual tests. *Br J Sports Med.* 2012;46(14):964-978.
11. Simão MN, Nogueira-Barbosa MH, Muglia VF, Barbieri CH. Anterior shoulder instability: Correlation between magnetic resonance arthrography, ultrasound arthrography and intraoperative findings. *Ultrasound Med Biol.* 2012;38(4):551-560.
12. Harwood MI, Smith CT. Superior labrum, anterior-posterior lesions and biceps injuries: Diagnostic and treatment considerations. *Prim Care.* 2004;31(4):831-855.
13. de Castro Pochini A, Ejnisman B, Andreoli CV, et al. Pectoralis major muscle rupture in athletes: A prospective study. *Am J Sports Med.* 2010;38(1):92-98.
14. Gillard J, Pérez-Cousin M, Hachulla E, et al. Diagnosing thoracic outlet syndrome: Contribution of provocative tests, ultrasonography, electrophysiology, and helical computed tomography in 48 patients. *Joint Bone Spine.* 2001;68(5):416-424.
15. Smith TO, Drew BT, Toms AP. A meta-analysis of the diagnostic test accuracy of MRA and MRI for the detection of glenoid labral injury. *Arch Orthop Trauma Surg.* 2012;132(7):905-919.
16. Rouleau DM, Hebert-Davies J. Incidence of associated injury in posterior shoulder dislocation: Systematic review of the literature. *J Orthop Trauma.* 2012;26(4):246-251.

17. Meister K, Buckley B, Batts J. The posterior impingement sign: Diagnosis of rotator cuff and posterior labral tears secondary to internal impingement in overhand athletes. *Am J Orthop (Belle Mead NJ).* 2004;33(8):412-415.
18. Tannenbaum E, Sekiya JK. Evaluation and management of posterior shoulder instability. *Sports Health.* 2011;3(3):253-263.
19. Forthomme B, Crielaard JM, Croisier JL. Scapular positioning in athlete's shoulder: Particularities, clinical measurements and implications. *Sports Med.* 2008;38(5):369-386.
20. Grieve R, Barnett S, Coghill N, Cramp F. The prevalence of latent myofascial trigger points and diagnostic criteria of the triceps surae and upper trapezius: A cross sectional study. *Physiotherapy.* 2013;99(4): 278-284.
21. Sewell MD, Al-Hadithy N, Le Leu A, Lambert SM. Instability of the sternoclavicular joint: Current concepts in classification, treatment and outcomes. *Bone Joint J.* 2013;95-B(6):721-731.
22. Rios CG, Mazzocca AD. Acromioclavicular joint problems in athletes and new methods of management. *Clin Sports Med.* 2008;27(4):763-788.
23. Robinson CM, Seah KT, Chee YH, Hindle P, Murray IR. Frozen shoulder. *J Bone Joint Surg Br.* 2012;94(1):1-9.
24. Feinberg JH, Radecki J. Parsonage-turner syndrome. *HSS J.* 2010 Sep;6(2):199-205.
25. Hegedus EJ, Goode A, Campbell S, et al. Physical examination tests of the shoulder: A systematic review with meta-analysis of individual tests. *Br J Sports Med.* 2008;42(2):80-92.

8

The Elbow

The elbow is a hinge joint that connects the distal humerus, proximal radius, and the ulna. The elbow region consists of three distinct articulations that must be considered: the lateral capitellum of the distal humerus articulates with the radial head, the trochlea of the humerus articulates with the proximal ulna, and the proximal radioulnar articulation. These joints work in concert to allow elbow flexion, extension, and forearm pronation and supination. The medial and lateral aspect of the elbow are supported by the medial (ulnar) and lateral (radial) collateral ligaments. These ligaments, in combination with the bony architecture, provide varus and valgus support. The elbow is particularly susceptible to medial instability based on the natural valgus carrying angle and the stresses placed on the elbow in overhead activities.

The muscles that cross the elbow and act on the wrist play a key role in some common elbow injuries. The flexor-pronator muscles that originate on the medial epicondyle of the humerus and the extensor-supinator muscles that originate on the lateral epicondyle of the humerus are frequently involved in overuse injures (epicondylitis), commonly referred to as golfer's and tennis elbow, respectively. The large biceps and triceps muscles allow for the elbow's primary movement of flexion and extension. The three main nerves of the forearm (ulnar, median, and radial) cross the elbow joint and are easily impacted by both trauma and overuse. The three major arteries associated with the elbow are the brachial, radial, and ulnar arteries. The brachial artery lies in the cubital fossa. Clinicians must be fully aware of the

Winterstein AP, Clark SV. *The Athletic Trainer's Guide to Differential Diagnosis (pp 239–271).*

location and function of these nerves and vessels when differentiating possible injuries; they take on added importance when contemplating traumatic injuries such as fracture and dislocation.

It is estimated that approximately 35 million children and adolescents participate in sports annually in the United States, and more than 2 million kids participate in Little League activities. Among children younger than 15 years, more than 3.5 million are treated for sports-related injuries. In particular, upper extremity and elbow injuries have increased, with 20% to 40% of 9- to 12-year-old baseball players and 50% to 70% of adolescent players developing elbow pain annually.[1] Injuries to the elbow take place in overhead throwing athletes as well as those who participate in weight bearing sports such as gymnastics. While fractures and dislocations commonly occur in collision sports and from falls, cartilage, subchondral bone, ligament, and apophyseal injuries occur from low-impact overuse activities.[2] Specific injuries in the growing child are different compared with injuries in adults, and this is even more pronounced in the skeletally immature elbow. Osteochondritis and other degenerative problems are not uncommon in this population.

Clinicians must be acutely aware of the range of possible acute and chronic elbow injuries in both adults and children. Knowledge of the underlying anatomy, coupled with an understanding of the variety of possible injuries, is essential when differentiating a diagnosis. Both students and practicing clinicians will be aided greatly by organizing their elbow evaluation using a diagnosis map.

Paper Patient: Elbow Pain in a Soccer Player

History

Robert is a 17-year-old soccer player who went up to head the ball during an away game and collided with another player, landing hard on his left elbow. He complained of significant elbow pain at the tip of his elbow at the time of injury; 2 days later, it has improved somewhat. He iced it right away, but there is still significant swelling in the elbow.

Physical Exam

On physical exam, the patient has tenderness over the olecranon on the left. The patient has pain with active motion from deep flexion to extension on the left. MMT for flexion and extension reveals pain greater for extension than flexion. Grip strength is 5/5 bilaterally. Ligamentous testing is negative. On observation, you do not see erythema, although there is deformity over the posterior elbow.

Clinical Decisions

Using the information from your clinical exam, ask yourself these questions to guide your clinical decision making:

- What is your differential diagnosis?
- What key findings do you see to help guide your differential?
- What are the possible injuries associated with posterior elbow pain?

Start with a review of the anatomy maps and a thorough consideration of the possible injuries and conditions that are common to the elbow. Use the differential diagnosis maps to guide your thought process and organize the possibilities. The organized synthesis of this information is the essence of clinical decision making. We will revisit this case at the end of the chapter.

Anatomy Map: Elbow

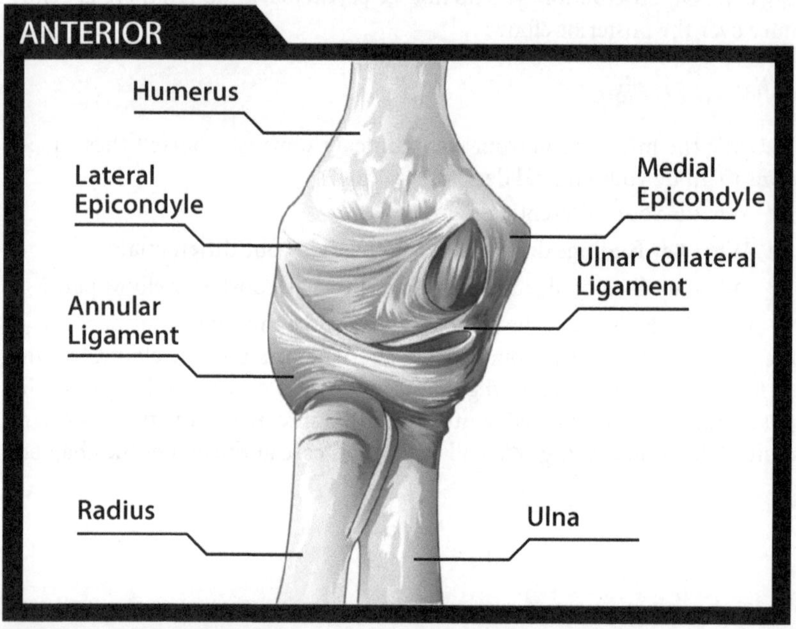

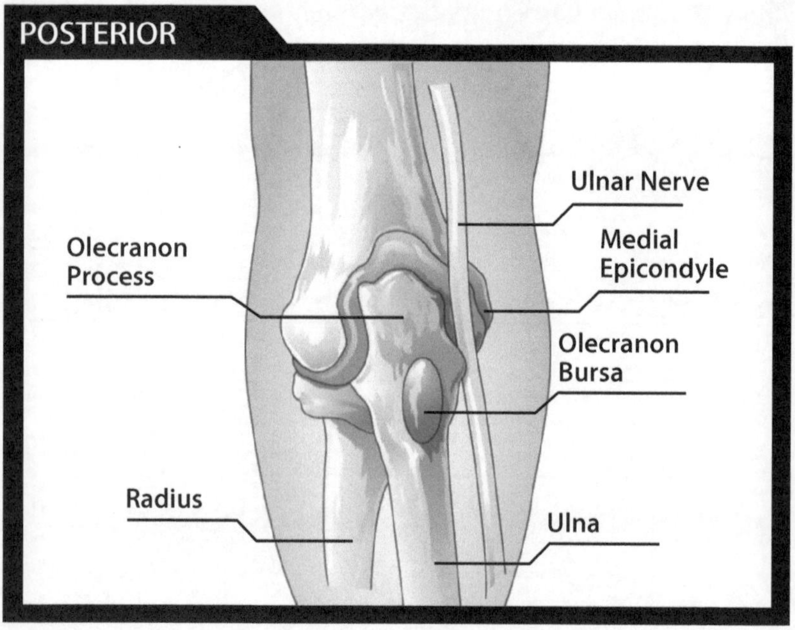

Anatomy Map: Elbow

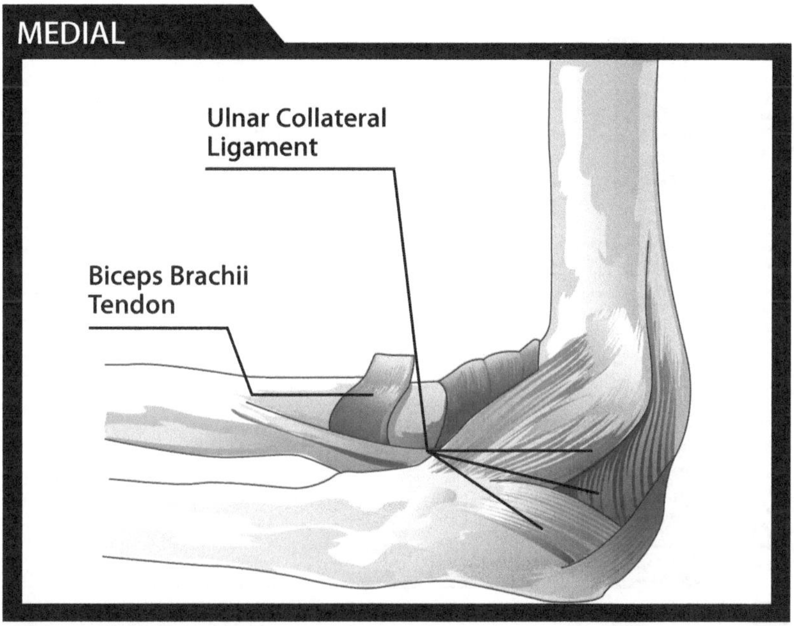

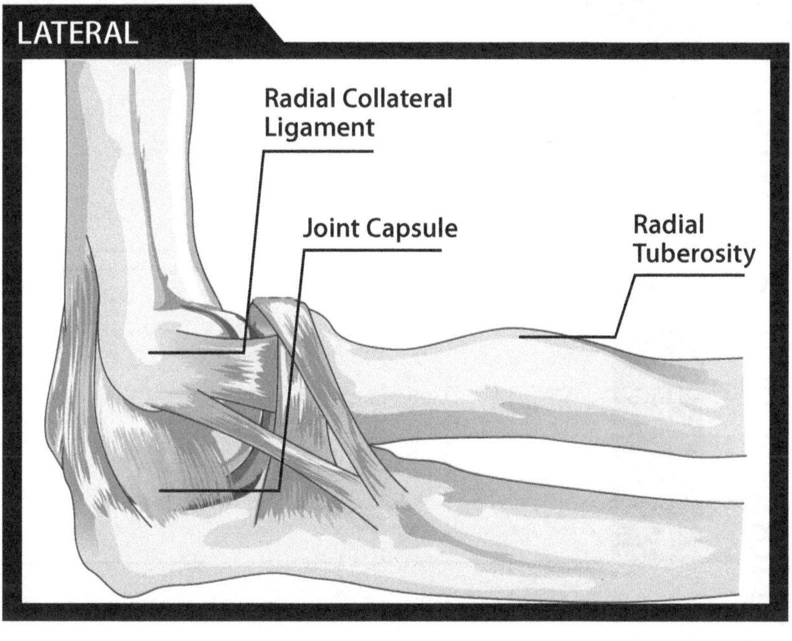

Elbow Pain Map: Region/Soft Tissue Differential Diagnosis

ANTERIOR

- Anterior Capsule Sprain/Climber's Elbow
- Anterior Dislocation
- Distal Biceps Tendinopathy
- Biceps Tendon Strain/Rupture
- Pronator Teres Syndrome

POSTERIOR

- Olecranon Bursitis
- Posterior Dislocation
- Triceps Rupture
- Triceps Strain
- Triceps Tendinopathy

MEDIAL

- Cubital Tunnel Syndrome
- Medial Apophysitis (Little League Elbow)
- Medial Dislocation
- Medial Epicondylitis
- Ulnar Collateral Ligament (UCL) Sprain

LATERAL

- Annular Ligament Sprain
- Forearm Compartment Syndrome
- Lateral Dislocation
- Lateral Epicondylitis
- Osteochondritis Dissecans
- Radial Collateral Ligament (RCL) Sprain
- Radial Head Dislocation
- Radial Nerve Injury

Elbow Pain

Injuries to Bone/Joint Surfaces

COMMON FRACTURES

- Lateral epicondyle fracture
- Medial epicondyle fracture
- Olecranon fracture
- Osteochondritis dissecans
- Arthroscopic Classification (Baumgarten)
    - Grade 1: Smooth but soft, ballotable articular cartilage
    - Grade 2: Fibrillations or fissuring of the cartilage
    - Grade 3: Exposed bone with a fixed osteochondral fragment
    - Grade 4: A loose but undisplaced fragment
    - Grade 5: A displaced fragment with resultant loose body
- Radial head dislocation
- Radial head fracture
- Radius shaft fracture
- Ulna fracture

Clinical Assessment of Elbow Injuries

Anterior Elbow Pain

Anterior Capsule Sprain/Climber's Elbow

HISTORY	MECHANISM OF INJURY	EVALUATION ESSENTIALS
• Pain and aching in the front of the elbow • Patient reports that the pain gets worse with a bent elbow against resistance and then trying to straighten elbow • The patient will have participated in one of the following activities: rock climbing, bowling, or pull ups	• Increase in training • Direct blow to the anterior elbow • Chronic repetitive elbow flexion • Forced extension/hyperextension	• Assess the brachialis muscle and there will be pain with this as well as crepitus • Inspect the anterior aspect for swelling • Evaluate muscle strength about the elbow

KEY FINDINGS	DIAGNOSTIC EVIDENCE
• The patient won't be able to fully straighten elbow • There will be crepitus when the tendon or elbow is moved or touched • There will be poor strength and flexibility	• No diagnostic evidence available

Anterior Elbow Pain

Anterior Dislocation

HISTORY	MECHANISM OF INJURY	EVALUATION ESSENTIALS
• Patient reports falling with arm flexed and a posterior force • Pain identified right away	• Fall resulting in a force striking the posterior forearm in a flexed position	• Assess the elbow with neurovascular tests • Inspect joint for deformity • Referral and radiographs necessary

KEY FINDINGS	DIAGNOSTIC EVIDENCE
• This is a rare dislocation that is usually accompanied by an olecranon fracture • Injury to nerve and blood vessel can occur frequently • The distal humerus is prominent posteriorly and the biceps tendon tents the skin anteriorly • The arm appears shortened and in supination	• Anterior dislocations only comprise approximately 15% of all dislocations and are often associated with complex fractures of the elbow and forearm[3]

Anterior Elbow Pain

Distal Biceps Tendinopathy

HISTORY	MECHANISM OF INJURY	EVALUATION ESSENTIALS
• Patient reports pain with palpation at the radial tuberosity • Pain identified with flexion and supination	• Sudden increase in activity • Repetitive supination and flexion	• Assess MMT for the biceps • Inspect the anterior elbow for swelling over the distal biceps tendon

KEY FINDINGS	DIAGNOSTIC EVIDENCE
• The patient will have pain with MMT of the biceps and possibly with supination of the wrist. • If tendinosis is acute the patient may present with swelling of the distal biceps • Crepitus may be present in acute cases	• MRI and ultrasound can be used to assist in diagnosis, but results are often inconclusive[4]

Anterior Elbow Pain

Biceps Tendon Strain/Rupture

HISTORY	MECHANISM OF INJURY	EVALUATION ESSENTIALS
• Patient reports a popping at the elbow • Pain identifies a defect in the muscle • The patient reports weakness at the elbow	• Acute when the elbow is forced straight against resistance, an eccentric load • Acute fall on an outstretched arm • May hear weight lifting in history	• Palpation of the entire biceps muscle • Assess muscle strength of the biceps to see if it is partially or fully torn

KEY FINDINGS	DIAGNOSTIC EVIDENCE
• May see ecchymosis • Inspection will reveal a defect in the biceps with a lump in the upper part of the arm if muscle has recoiled • The patient will be weak or have difficulty contracting biceps	• Three special tests have been found to have 100% sensitivity and specificity for a distal biceps tendon rupture in comparison to MRI: hook test, passive forearm pronation, and biceps crease interval[5]

Anterior Elbow Pain

Pronator Teres Syndrome

HISTORY	MECHANISM OF INJURY	EVALUATION ESSENTIALS
• The patient complains of numbness, tingling, and/or a pins and needles sensation in thumb, index finger, middle finger, and half the ring finger • Patient reports having trouble gripping and turning wrist over	• Edema over the pronator teres causing entrapment of the median nerve • Hypertrophy of the pronator teres muscle can cause entrapment of the median nerve • Chronic repetitive pronation at the wrist	• Test RROM for pronation and elbow flexion • Assess upper limb nerve tension for median nerve • Inspect for atrophy of the forearm flexor group • Tinel's sign, Phalen's, and reverse Phalen's sign

KEY FINDINGS	DIAGNOSTIC EVIDENCE
• Differential between carpal tunnel syndrome and pronator teres syndrome is the location of the median nerve compression (at or near elbow in pronator teres syndrome) • Weakness in grip strength and difficulty putting thumb and index finger together • Upper limb nerve tension testing may elicit symptoms in the elbow area • MMT will reproduce symptoms	• Electrodiagnostic testing can assist in diagnosis • Many special tests are mentioned in the literature but sensitivity and specificity have not been reported[6]

Posterior Elbow Pain

Olecranon Bursitis

HISTORY	MECHANISM OF INJURY	EVALUATION ESSENTIALS
• Patient reports swelling over the posterior elbow • Pain identified pain over the posterior elbow	• Direct trauma to the olecranon • Prolonged pressure on the tip of the elbow • Infection	• Observe posterior elbow for swelling and erythema • Palpate for warmth • Assess patient for infection • Evaluate muscle strength

KEY FINDINGS	DIAGNOSTIC EVIDENCE
• The patient will be point tender over the olecranon • May see erythema • Olecranon may be warm to the touch • Swelling can be severe	• Radiographs may be indicated for acute trauma to rule out olecranon fracture, but are not performed routinely for this condition[7]

Posterior Elbow Pain

Posterior Dislocation

HISTORY	MECHANISM OF INJURY	EVALUATION ESSENTIALS
• Patient reports falling on an outstretched arm • Acute onset of pain • Immediate loss of function	• FOOSH mechanism with elbow in extension on impact	• Assess the elbow with neurovascular tests • Inspect joint for deformity • Referral and radiographs necessary

KEY FINDINGS	DIAGNOSTIC EVIDENCE
• This is the most common of the elbow dislocations • Injury to nerve and blood vessel can occur frequently • Will potentially find the patient to be pulseless • The arm appears shortened in flexion with posterior prominence	• Radiographs or CT are used to determine if there are associated fractures[8]

Posterior Elbow Pain

Triceps Rupture

HISTORY	MECHANISM OF INJURY	EVALUATION ESSENTIALS
• Patient reports painful pop at the elbow • Pain identified at the posterior elbow	• Forceful eccentric contraction • Fall on an outstretched arm	• Assess ROM against gravity • Palpation of the distal triceps for defect • Inspect for swelling and ecchymosis

KEY FINDINGS	DIAGNOSTIC EVIDENCE
• The patient will have a defect at the triceps most likely the medial or lateral head • The patient will demonstrate a loss of ability to extend elbow against gravity • The patient will have swelling and/or ecchymosis depending upon the timing of the exam	• MRI can be used to determine whether it was a partial or full rupture • Studies have shown an increased incidence of triceps tendon ruptures after receiving corticosteroid injections for olecranon bursitis[9]

Posterior Elbow Pain

Triceps Strain

HISTORY	MECHANISM OF INJURY	EVALUATION ESSENTIALS
• Patient reports pain at rest and during activity • Pain identified at the posterior elbow	• Overuse injury (eg, weight lifting) • Repetitive elbow extension • Tissue overload (eg, pushing something that is too heavy)	• Assess RROM for the triceps • Palpation of the distal triceps • Evaluate AROM and PROM

KEY FINDINGS	DIAGNOSTIC EVIDENCE
• The patient will have pain at the triceps insertion • The patient will have limited mobility depending upon severity of the strain • The patient will have pain with extension and against resisted extension	• Severity of the strain can be evaluated by MRI, but is not considered standard of care[10]

Posterior Elbow Pain

Triceps Tendinopathy

HISTORY	MECHANISM OF INJURY	EVALUATION ESSENTIALS
• Patient reports pain at the posterior elbow • The patient may complain of crepitus with motion of the elbow	• Acutely with forceful eccentric contraction typically with weight lifting • May be chronic with repetitive pushing activity	• Assess AROM and PROM • Palpation of the distal triceps for pain • Inspect for swelling • MMT of the triceps

KEY FINDINGS	DIAGNOSTIC EVIDENCE
• The patient will have pain at the triceps distally • The patient will demonstrate weakness and/or pain with MMT of the triceps • The patient will have swelling if severe tendinosis	• Ultrasound and MRI can help detect changes in the tendon[11]

Medial Elbow Pain

Cubital Tunnel Syndrome

HISTORY	MECHANISM OF INJURY	EVALUATION ESSENTIALS
• Patient complains of radiating medial elbow pain • Patient may experience tingling the fourth and fifth fingers • May wake with tingling in the last two fingers • Pain identified with elbow hyperflexion	• Pronounced cubitus valgus creating friction or subluxing of ulnar nerve • Ulnar nerve irritation with repetitive flexion activity • Traction injury from a valgus force • Irregularities in the tunnel	• Assess throwing mechanics if appropriate • Identify elbow posture in anatomical position • Tinel's test over ulnar nerve • Perform AROM and PROM testing • Evaluate muscle strength

KEY FINDINGS	DIAGNOSTIC EVIDENCE
• The patient will likely present with a valgus deformity • Patient will experience a popping with flexion and extension of the elbow • The patient will experience burning and/or tingling in the fourth and fifth fingers • The patient may note a change in sensation	• History and physical examination alone are often enough to diagnosis this syndrome, but electrodiagnostic testing may be used for confirmation[12]

Medial Elbow Pain

Medial Aphophysitis (Little League Elbow)

HISTORY	MECHANISM OF INJURY	EVALUATION ESSENTIALS
• Patient reports catching or locking and decreased motion of the elbow • Chronic slow onset • Pain identified with throwing	• Abnormal stresses to the elbow from volume of throwing (regardless of kind of pitch thrown) • Repetitive poor throwing mechanics	• Measure ROM at the elbow • Assess AROM and PROM • Inspect elbow joint and palpate • Evaluate muscle strength

KEY FINDINGS	DIAGNOSTIC EVIDENCE
• The patient will have weakness of the triceps • There will be a complaint of catching or locking • The patient has a flexion contracture or complains of tightening of the anterior elbow • There is decreased pronation and supination	• Radiographs and MRI may be used to determine if there is physeal damage, osteochondritis dissecans, or early arthritis[13]

Medial Elbow Pain

Medial Dislocation

HISTORY	MECHANISM OF INJURY	EVALUATION ESSENTIALS
• Patient reports falling on an outstretched arm • Pain identified right away	• Acute trauma with a valgus force • Fall with elbow in partial flexion and valgus position • FOOSH mechanism with elbow in extension with rotation on impact	• Assess the elbow with neurovascular tests • Inspect joint for deformity • Referral and radiographs necessary

KEY FINDINGS	DIAGNOSTIC EVIDENCE
• This is a rare dislocation of the elbow • Injury to nerve and blood vessel can occur frequently • The arm appears with medial elbow prominence	• Medial elbow dislocations often result in instability and may need further imaging to determine the amount of soft tissue damage and need for surgery[14]

Medial Elbow Pain

Medial Epicondylitis

HISTORY	MECHANISM OF INJURY	EVALUATION ESSENTIALS
• Patient reports pain at the medial elbow potentially radiating down the arm • Pain identified with active motion at the elbow and wrist as well as with gripping	• Poor mechanics with golf, tennis, swimming, or rowing • Chronic overuse of the wrist flexors • Overdoing activities such as painting, hammering, or using a screw driver	• Assess AROM and PROM • Inspect medial elbow for swelling • Evaluate muscle strength through resisted flexion and pronation

KEY FINDINGS	DIAGNOSTIC EVIDENCE
• Pain starts off as sporadic and progresses to constant in severe cases • May see swelling if severe • Pain with resisted wrist flexion and pronation; pain will not likely be with passive motion, rather active and resisted	• Imaging is only used when conservative treatment fails • Ultrasound (sensitivity 64% to 82%) • MRI (sensitivity 90% to 100%)[15]

Medial Elbow Pain

Ulnar Collateral Ligament Sprain

HISTORY	MECHANISM OF INJURY	EVALUATION ESSENTIALS
• Patient reports a fall or repetitive throwing • Patient describes a stiffness and pain (with activities) in elbow • Patient is unable to throw at full speed, has loss of control, and weak grip	• Sudden FOOSH • Improper throwing mechanics • Repetitive stress from throwing	• Perform AROM and PROM • Assess valgus stress testing at 0 and 20 to 30 degrees of elbow flexion • Inspect for swelling and ecchymosis • Evaluate muscle strength

KEY FINDINGS	DIAGNOSTIC EVIDENCE
• The patient will have a positive valgus stress test • Patient will report pop or pulling sensation at the time of injury depending upon severity of injury • Patient without full extension motion at the elbow • May see ecchymosis and swelling depending upon the timing of the exam • The patient will have decreased grip strength and weakness with MMT	• MRI for full thickness tears (sensitivity 100%, specificity 100%) • MRI for partial thickness tears (sensitivity 57%, specificity 100%)[16] • Tenderness over the UCL (sensitivity 81% to 94%, specificity 22%) • Valgus stress test (sensitivity 66%, specificity 60%)[17]

Lateral Elbow Pain

Annular Ligament Sprain

HISTORY	MECHANISM OF INJURY	EVALUATION ESSENTIALS
• Patient reports pain over the lateral elbow and into the hand • Pain identified with throwing, forehand in tennis, or any rotation activity	• High demand forces from sports that require throwing with rotation • Improper stretching and throwing mechanics that could stem from year round sport participation in softball or baseball	• Assess laxity of the annular ligament • Palpation of the deep annular ligament • Evaluate muscle strength

KEY FINDINGS	DIAGNOSTIC EVIDENCE
• Pain is elicited with palpation of the lateral epicondyle and worse over the annular ligament • The patient will experience pain that radiates to the thumb, index, and middle finger just as in carpal tunnel syndrome • Often misdiagnosed as lateral epicondylitis	• MRI is the most accurate diagnostic test for assessing the annular ligament[18]

Lateral Elbow Pain

Forearm Compartment Syndrome

HISTORY	MECHANISM OF INJURY	EVALUATION ESSENTIALS
• Patient reports pain in forearm with activity and better without activity • Pain also identified with no activity depending upon mechanism	• Secondary complication from fractures most common • From tight cast or other compressive dressing • Any arterial injury, bleeding disorder, or excessive swelling • Crush injury/contusions • From a gunshot wound	• Assess AROM and PROM • Check pulse and nerve testing • Inspect forearm for bleeding, swelling, ecchymosis • Evaluate muscle strength • Refer for radiograph to rule out fracture and pressure testing

KEY FINDINGS	DIAGNOSTIC EVIDENCE
• The patient will have increased pain with active motion or muscle testing of the forearm • Pain out of proportion to activity • Patient may have paresthesia or hypoesthesia, and lack peripheral pulses depending upon severity and timing of exam • The history will match the physical exam findings such as history of crush injury	• Most common cause of forearm compartment syndrome in adults is a distal radial fracture; therefore radiographs are required to help determine the source of symptoms • Intra-compartmental pressure testing is often completed to confirm diagnosis • Sensory deficits are reported as the most common symptom[19]

Lateral Elbow Pain

Lateral Dislocation

HISTORY	MECHANISM OF INJURY	EVALUATION ESSENTIALS
• Patient reports falling on an outstretched arm • Pain identified right away	• FOOSH mechanism with elbow in extension with rotation/varus position on impact	• Assess the elbow with neurovascular tests • Inspect joint for deformity • Referral and radiographs necessary

KEY FINDINGS	DIAGNOSTIC EVIDENCE
• This is a rare dislocation of the elbow • Injury to nerve and blood vessel can occur frequently • The arm appears with lateral elbow prominence	• Only several cases have been reported in the literature with an estimated incidence of 0.7% • Radiographs imperative for accurate assessment[20]

Lateral Elbow Pain

Lateral Epicondylitis

HISTORY	MECHANISM OF INJURY	EVALUATION ESSENTIALS
• Patient reports pain at the lateral elbow • Pain identified with gripping and with wrist extension	• Repetitive overuse of the forearm extensors chronic • After a full day of repetitive activity such as chopping wood • With racquet sports, the backhand stroke is most provoking	• Palpate the lateral epicondyle • Assess MMT and motion wrist extension, pronation, supination, and grip • Inspect for swelling and tissue tension over lateral elbow • Check biomechanics and shoulder strength

KEY FINDINGS	DIAGNOSTIC EVIDENCE
• There will be pain at the lateral epicondyle • Tissue tension noted throughout the extensor mass • Pain with gripping • Pain with MMT for the wrist extensors, pronators and supinators at 0 and/or 90 degrees of elbow flexion	• Imaging is only used when conservative treatment fails • Ultrasound (sensitivity 64% to 82%) • MRI (sensitivity 90% to 100%)[15]

Lateral Elbow Pain

Osteochondritis Dissecans

HISTORY

- Patient will be preteen or in early to mid teens (10 to 15 years old)
- Patient reports lateral elbow pain and locking
- Chronic onset
- Pain identified with throwing or racquet sports

MECHANISM OF INJURY

- Repetitive elbow extension, rotation, and valgus stress
- May be a traumatic origin
- Valgus instability and overuse can cause compression on lateral aspect of the elbow

EVALUATION ESSENTIALS

- Assess AROM and PROM
- Assess for valgus instability
- Refer and radiograph
- Evaluate muscle strength

KEY FINDINGS

- There is dull, aching, persistent pain at the elbow
- There will be capitellar deformity
- Osteochondrosis of the capitellum is also called Panner's disease
- There will be loose fragments found on radiograph and there will be uptake on subchondral bone in the capitellum

DIAGNOSTIC EVIDENCE

- Radiographs and MRI are often used for evaluation, but their accuracy is debated in the literature
- Arthroscopy is often considered the gold standard for evaluating the instability of OCD fragments[21]
- Radiographs can identify Panner's disease, but MRI is considered more sensitive for assessment of the capitellum[22]

Lateral Elbow Pain

Radial Collateral Ligament (RCL) Sprain

HISTORY	MECHANISM OF INJURY	EVALUATION ESSENTIALS
• Patient reports pain at the lateral elbow • Patient complains of mechanical symptoms such as clicking and catching with elbow extension • Pain identified with pushing up from a chair	• Traumatic seen with dislocation • May be seen as a complication from surgery to the lateral elbow • May be secondary to chronic cubits varus malunion	• Varus testing at the elbow • Assess lateral pivot shift test • Palpation of the RCL • May need to refer for radiograph if trauma is mechanism • Evaluate muscle strength

KEY FINDINGS	DIAGNOSTIC EVIDENCE
• The patient will have laxity with varus and pivot shift testing • The patient will have pain and mechanical symptoms with pushing up from a chair • The patient will have pain with palpation of the lateral elbow over the RCL	• The pivot shift test and the push-up from a chair test have a reported sensitivity of 87% alone and 100% when combined[25]

Lateral Elbow Pain

Radial Head Dislocation

HISTORY	MECHANISM OF INJURY	EVALUATION ESSENTIALS
• Patient reports pain at the elbow • Will either be acute or chronic depending upon patient and history • Pain identified with motion at the elbow	• Traumatic injury dislocates radial head anteriorly • Fall on outstretched, pronated arm • Result of cerebral palsy or neurological injury the radial head will dislocate posterolaterally • Congenital disorder radial head dislocates posteriorly and is often bilateral • Ehler's Danlos syndrome	• Assess AROM and PROM • Inspect radial head • Refer and radiograph • Evaluate muscle strength

KEY FINDINGS	DIAGNOSTIC EVIDENCE
• The acute mechanism will have a history to go with the physical exam and likewise for the non traumatic case which will likely be bilateral • Observable deformity • Younger patients will likely have a subluxation and history of being grabbed at the wrist to swing or pick up child by the arm	• Radiographs are not considered necessary if clinical presentation is consistent with a radial head dislocation • First attempt reduction rates are high (~95%)[23]

Lateral Elbow Pain

Radial Nerve Injury

HISTORY	MECHANISM OF INJURY	EVALUATION ESSENTIALS
• The patient reports pain in the forearm • Patient reports burning or numbness and tingling • Pain identified with repetitive forearm pronation	• Compression of the radial nerve • May be from blow to lateral elbow • Repetitive pronation and supination	• Check Tinel's tap test over the radial nerve • Upper limb nerve tension test for the radial nerve • Assess the upper quarter screen • Evaluate muscle strength

KEY FINDINGS	DIAGNOSTIC EVIDENCE
• The patient will have a positive upper limb nerve tension test for the radial nerve • Positive Tinel's tap test • Pain to palpation over the radial nerve • General hand weakness • There will be weakness of wrist and finger extension	• Imaging and electrodiagnostic testing are often inconclusive • The use of an injected local anesthetic can help differentiate from lateral epicondylitis[24]

Paper Patient: Revisited

You should have been able to rule out several conditions secondary to knowing what structures are at the posterior elbow. Your differential diagnosis for the case presented at the start of the chapter should have been olecranon bursitis versus fracture.

Learning Activities: Practice Case

Use the blank templates provided in the Appendices to write out a differential diagnosis map and clinical findings overview for the case provided below. When working with paper patients, it is tempting to try to jump to "the answer" and come to a diagnosis. However, the visual learning approach to differential diagnosis is designed to help you consider all the possibilities for the information provided. Good luck.

Paper Patient: Elbow Pain in a Middle-Aged Man

History

Fred is a 50-year-old attorney who reports right lateral elbow pain when using his mouse at work. He plays guitar for 1 hour a day, 5 times per week, and his pain is with strumming. He plays piano for 1 to 1.5 hours per day and this is painful. He gardens regularly and has pain right now with the shovel work. He denies any history of neck pain or previous injury to the elbow. He has pain with some activities of daily living but not all. For instance, he can pull the covers up in bed or grab a gallon of milk from the refrigerator without pain, but he has pain with turning doorknobs.

Physical Exam

On physical exam, the patient has tenderness to palpation at the lateral epicondyle and extensor mass. The extensor mass is tight compared to the left side with palpation. He has pain with MMT with extension of the wrist as well as pronation and supination. Resisted extension of the third digit reproduces pain at the lateral elbow. MMT of the brachialis is negative for pain, and the brachioradialis is positive for pain. Strength is limited by pain. His upper limb nerve tension tests are positive for both the radial and median nerves.

References

1. Ireland ML, Hutchinson MR. Upper extremity injuries in young athletes. *Clin Sports Med.* 1995;14(3):533-569.
2. Greiwe MR, Comron S, Ahmad CS. Pediatric sports elbow injuries. *Clin Sports Med.* 2010;29(4):677-703.
3. de Haan J, Schep N, Tuinebreijer W, den Hartog D. Complex and unstable simple elbow dislocations: A review and quantitative analysis of individual patient data. *Open Orthop J.* 2010;4:80-86.
4. Hobbs MC, Koch J, Bamberger HB. Distal biceps tendinosis: Evidence-based review. *J Hand Surg Am.* 2009;34(6):1124-1126.
5. Devereaux MW, ElMaraghy AW. Improving the rapid and reliable diagnosis of complete distal biceps tendon rupture: A nuanced approach to the clinical examination. *Am J Sports Med.* 2013;41(9):1998-2004.
6. Presciutti S, Rodner CM. Pronator syndrome. *J Hand Surg Am.* 2011;36(5):907-909.
7. Del Buono A, Franceschi F, Palumbo A, Denaro V, Maffulli N. Diagnosis and management of olecranon bursitis. *Surgeon.* 2012;10(5):297-300.
8. McCabe MP, Savoie FH 3rd. Simple elbow dislocations: Evaluation, management, and outcomes. *Phys Sportsmed.* 2012;40(1):62-71.
9. Rineer CA, Ruch DS. Elbow tendinopathy and tendon ruptures: Epicondylitis, biceps and triceps ruptures. *J Hand Surg Am.* 2009;34(3):566-576.
10. Koplas MC, Schneider E, Sundaram M. Prevalence of triceps tendon tears on MRI of the elbow and clinical correlation. *Skeletal Radiol.* 2011;40(5):587-594.
11. Fedorczyk JM. Tendinopathies of the elbow, wrist, and hand: Histopathology and clinical considerations. *J Hand Ther.* 2012;25(2):191-200.
12. Kroonen LT. Cubital tunnel syndrome. *Orthop Clin North Am.* 2012;43(4):475-486.
13. Wei AS, Khana S, Limpisvasti O, Crues J, Podesta L, Yocum LA. Clinical and magnetic resonance imaging findings associated with Little League elbow. *J Pediatr Orthop.* 2010;30(7):715-719.
14. Jockel CR, Katolik LI, Zelouf DS. Simple medial elbow dislocations: A rare injury at risk for early instability. *J Hand Surg Am.* 2013;38(9):1768-1773.
15. Walz DM, Newman JS, Konin GP, Ross G. Epicondylitis: Pathogenesis, imaging, and treatment. *Radiographics.* 2010;30(1):167-184.
16. Kijowski R, Tuite M, Sanford M. Magnetic resonance imaging of the elbow. Part II: Abnormalities of the ligaments, tendons, and nerves. *Skeletal Radiol.* 2005;34(1):1-18.
17. Hariri S, Safran MR. Ulnar collateral ligament injury in the overhead athlete. *Clin Sports Med.* 2010;29(4):619-644.
18. Husarik DB, Saupe N, Pfirrmann CW, Jost B, Hodler J, Zanetti M. Ligaments and plicae of the elbow: Normal MR imaging variability in 60 asymptomatic subjects. *Radiology.* 2010;257(1):185-194.
19. Kalyani BS, Fisher BE, Roberts CS, Giannoudis PV. Compartment syndrome of the forearm: A systematic review. *J Hand Surg Am.* 2011;36(3):535-543.
20. Zaraa M, Saied W, Bouchoucha S, Ben Ghachem M. [Purely lateral elbow dislocation in a child, case report and literature review]. *Chir Main.* 2012;31(1):38-40.
21. Heywood CS, Benke MT, Brindle K, Fine KM. Correlation of magnetic resonance imaging to arthroscopic findings of stability in juvenile osteochondritis dissecans. *Arthroscopy.* 2011;27(2):194-199.
22. Stoane JM, Poplausky MR, Haller JO, Berdon WE. Panner's disease: X-ray, MR imaging findings and review of the literature. *Comput Med Imaging Graph.* 1995;19(6):473-476.

23. Lavallee ME, Sears K, Corrigan A. The evaluation and treatment of elbow injuries. *Prim Care.* 2013;40(2):407-429.
24. Naam NH, Nemani S. Radial tunnel syndrome. *Orthop Clin North Am.* 2012;43(4):529-536.
25. Reichel LM, Milam GS, Sitton SE, Curry MC, Mehlhoff TL. Elbow lateral collateral ligament injuries. *J Hand Surg Am.* 2013;38(1):184-201.

9

The Wrist and Hand

The hand and wrist are commonly injured in sport and physical activity. Rettig[1] found that between 3% and 9% of all sports injuries involve the hand and wrist. Hand and wrist injuries can be divided into two major classifications: traumatic and overuse. Traumatic injuries include fractures, dislocations, and ligament tears often seen in contact/collision sports. Stress and overuse conditions are frequently seen in gymnastics, racquet sports, and golf.[1,2] Swensen et al[3] surveyed sports-related injuries in high school athletes and found that the hand and wrist were the most common body regions injured, accounting for 40% of all fractures. The most common athletic fracture in the wrist is the carpal scaphoid fracture, which accounts for 70% of all carpal fractures.[4] The scaphoid fracture is most prevalent in the 15- to 30-year-old population. By their very nature, sports require repetitive grabbing, catching, and throwing of objects; this coupled with the frequency of the FOOSH mechanism of injury make it easy to see why there are a wide variety of traumatic and overuse injuries to the hand and wrist. Hand and wrist injuries are also common in extreme sport activities; finger tendon injures are common among rock climbers.[5]

The wrist serves to position the hand for a variety of gripping and grasping actions. Knowledge of underlying anatomy is critical to thorough evaluation of the wrist and hand, and for differentiating the proper diagnosis. Although the anatomy of the wrist and hand is complex, the superficial location of the majority of structures makes direct palpation possible and enhances the ability of the clinician to establish a diagnosis. As sport

Winterstein AP, Clark SV. *The Athletic Trainer's Guide to Differential Diagnosis (pp 273–320).*

participation rates rise among children and adolescents, and the Baby Boom generation stays active longer, clinicians will need to be well informed on injuries to the wrist and hand to properly diagnose and establish treatment plans.[6] Two differential diagnosis maps are provided in this chapter to aid in mapping injuries to the wrist and hand. The maps are divided into medial, lateral, dorsal, and palmar regions. Separate injuries are mapped for the fingers and the thumb. Students and clinicians should use these maps to delineate both acute and overuse injuries to the wrist and hand.

Paper Patient: Thumb Pain in a Rock Climber

History

Jolene is a 48-year-old right-handed female who comes to your clinic complaining of pain in her left thumb and hand. She is an avid rock climber in her free time and an administrative assistant by day. She reports that the pain has been going on for the past month and it has been getting worse. She has noticed that she doesn't seem to have the same strength when climbing lately and that concerns her more than the pain.

Physical Exam

Your physical exam reveals tenderness to palpation over the hand, mostly the thumb, index finger, and into the palm. There is pain with active motion on the left for flexion and extension of the wrist. The patient has a loss of grip strength on the left as compared to the right. The patient complains of numbness and tingling into her thumb and index finger on the left and not the right during palpation. Strength is 4/5 for thumb abduction left and 5/5 for right. Ligamentous testing is negative. Finkelstein's test is negative. The patient has positive Tinel's tap test over the median nerve and nerve tension testing of the median nerve.

Clinical Decisions

Using the information from your clinical exam, ask yourself these questions to guide your clinical decision making:

- What is your differential diagnosis?
- What key findings do you see to help guide your differential?
- What are the possible injuries associated with thumb and hand pain?

Start with a review of the anatomy maps and a thorough consideration of the possible injuries and conditions that are common to the wrist and hand. Use the differential diagnosis maps to guide your thought process and organize the possibilities. The organized synthesis of this information is the essence of clinical decision making. We will revisit this case at the end of the chapter.

Anatomy Map: Wrist

ANTERIOR

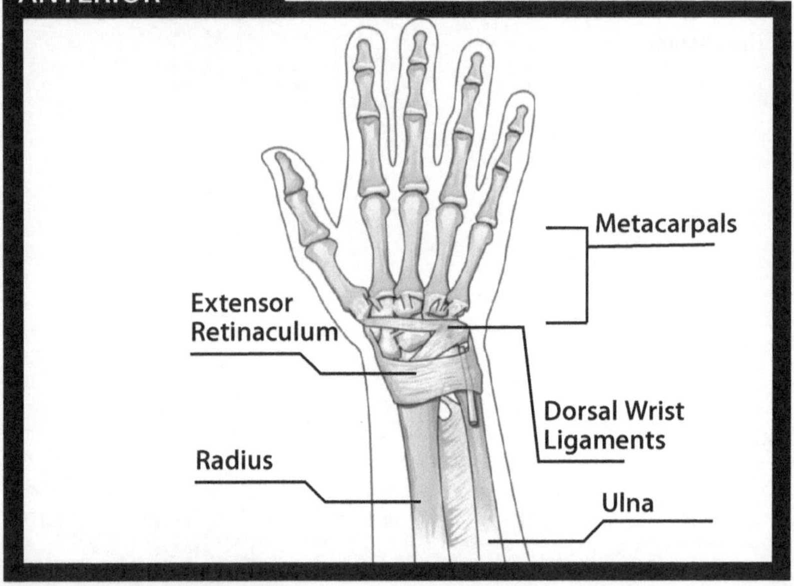

PALMAR

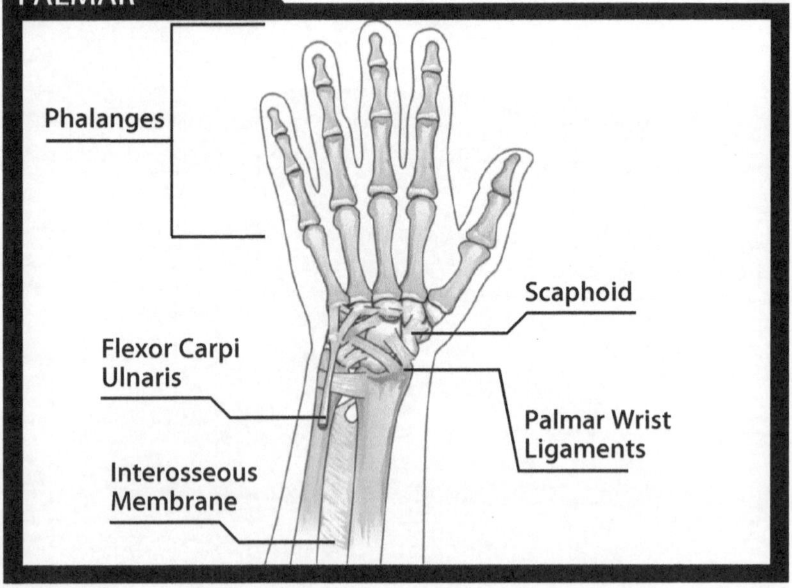

Anatomy Map: Wrist

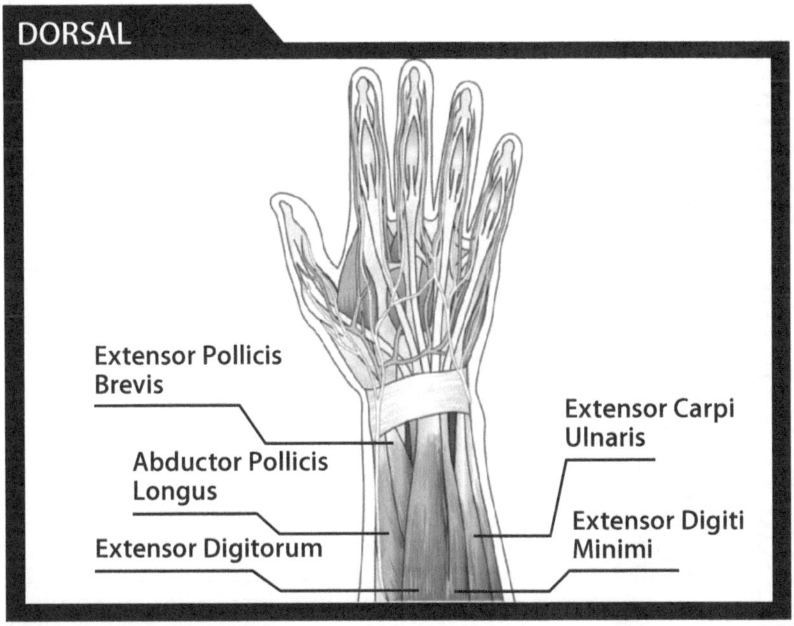

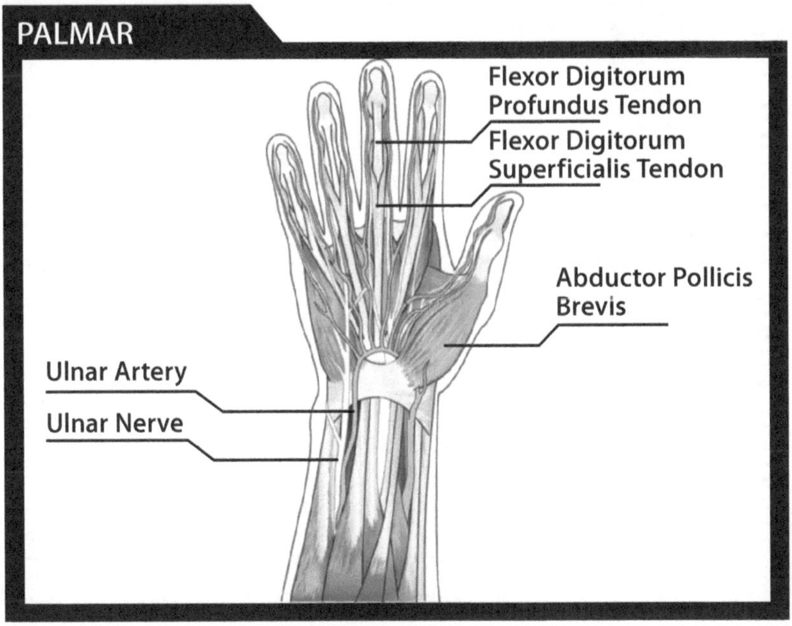

Wrist Map: Region/Soft Tissue Differential Diagnosis

PALMAR

- Carpal Tunnel Syndrome
- Flexor Tendinopathy
- Median and Ulnar Nerve Injury (Claw Hand)
- Median Nerve Injury (Ape Hand Deformity)
- Radiocarpal Ligament Sprain
- Ulnocarpal Ligament Sprain

DORSAL

- Extensor Tendinopathy
- Ganglion Cyst
- Lunate Dislocation
- Radial Nerve Injury (Drop-Wrist Deformity)
- Radiocarpal Ligament Sprain
- Ulnocarpal Ligament Sprain

ULNAR

- Triangular Fibrocartilage Complex (TFCC) Injury
- Ulnar Collateral Ligament Sprain
- Ulnar Nerve Injury (Benediction or Bishop's Deformity)

RADIAL

- Radial Collateral Ligament Sprain

Wrist and Hand Injury

Injuries to Bone/Joint Surfaces

COMMON FRACTURES

- Wrist
    - First metacarpal into CMC joint (Bennett's)
    - Fifth metacarpal (Boxer's)
    - Avulsion of flexor/extensor tendons
    - Carpals
        - Hook of the hamate
        - Scaphoid
    - Distal radius
    - Distal radius with dorsal displacement (Colles')
    - Distal radius with palmar displacement (Smith's)
    - Distal ulna
- Hand
    - Distal phalanx
    - Metacarpal
    - Phalanges
        - Distal phalanx
        - Middle phalanx
        - Proximal phalanx

Clinical Assessment of Wrist Injuries

Palmar Wrist Pain

Carpal Tunnel Syndrome

HISTORY	MECHANISM OF INJURY	EVALUATION ESSENTIALS
• Patient reports dropping things • Patient complains of weakness in the thumb and possibly numbness and tingling in the hand • Pain identified with typing or using a mouse	• Compression of the median nerve secondary to tenosynovitis of the flexor tendons • Complication of diabetes or alcoholism • Chronic describe nature (eg, repetitive impact)	• Assess AROM and PROM • Inspect and palpate hand • Upper limb nerve tension test for the median nerve • Phalen's, reverse Phalen's, and Tinel's • May refer for nerve conduction and EMG testing • MMT

KEY FINDINGS	DIAGNOSTIC EVIDENCE
• Patient will have positive Phalen's, reverse Phalen's, and upper limb nerve tension test for the median nerve • Patient will have decreased sensation in the hand at the median nerve distribution • Patient will have weakness into the thumb and possibly atrophy of the thenar eminence if prolonged symptoms	• Phalen's test (sensitivity 46% to 80%, specificity 51% to 91%) • Tinel's test (sensitivity 28 to 73%, specificity 44% to 95%)[7]

Palmar Wrist Pain

Flexor Tendinopathy

HISTORY	MECHANISM OF INJURY	EVALUATION ESSENTIALS
• Patient reports aching and stiffness in wrist and hand • Gradual onset • Patient complains of pain with ADLs as time goes on	• Repetitive or forceful gripping or use of flexors • Sudden increase in activities involving the hand • Possibly traumatic due to a fall	• Assess AROM and PROM • Inspect and palpate wrist and hand • Evaluate muscle strength in the wrist and hand

KEY FINDINGS	DIAGNOSTIC EVIDENCE
• Patient will have pain with wrist flexor testing • Patients may have pins and needles feeling or numbness in the hand • Patient will have pain and reduced strength with gripping	• Diagnosis is often by physical examination alone, but MRI and ultrasonography can be used to evaluate integrity of the tendons

Palmar Wrist Pain

Median and Ulnar Nerve Injury (Claw Hand)

HISTORY	MECHANISM OF INJURY	EVALUATION ESSENTIALS
• Patient reports not being able to extend wrist or fingers • Pain is described as sharp and burning	• Direct trauma to the nerve • Compression of the ulnar and median nerve	• Assess AROM and PROM • Inspect wrist and hand • Evaluate muscle strength

KEY FINDINGS	DIAGNOSTIC EVIDENCE
• There is paralysis of the extensors of all digits, all fingers including the thumb are in a flexed and extended position • The patient may have sharp and severe pain	• Electrodiagnostic testing may be used to confirm diagnosis[7]

Palmar Wrist Pain

Median Nerve Injury (Ape Hand Deformity)

HISTORY	MECHANISM OF INJURY	EVALUATION ESSENTIALS
• Patient reports not being able to use the thumb away from the remaining fingers • Patient complains of weakness in the thumb	• Laceration at the wrist • Possibly from supracondylar fracture of humerus • Compression of the median nerve secondary to trauma creating a palsy	• Assess AROM and PROM • Inspect and palpate hand • Refer for nerve conduction and EMG testing • Evaluate muscle strength in the hand

KEY FINDINGS	DIAGNOSTIC EVIDENCE
• Patient will have an inability to abduct the thumb • Patients thumb will be pulled backward by the extensor muscles • Patient will lose ability to grip	• Electrodiagnostic testing may be used to confirm diagnosis • Radiographs and MRI may be used to determine source of symptoms[7]

Palmar Wrist Pain

Radiocarpal Ligament Sprain

HISTORY	MECHANISM OF INJURY	EVALUATION ESSENTIALS
• Patient reports pain and swelling and difficulty moving the wrist • Patient complains of pain on the radial side of the wrist	• Abnormal or forced movement at the wrist • Possibly traumatic due to a fall with wrist extended	• Assess AROM and PROM • Inspect wrist for swelling and palpate wrist for tenderness • Evaluate muscle strength in the wrist

KEY FINDINGS	DIAGNOSTIC EVIDENCE
• Patient will have pain with wrist flexor testing • Patients will likely have swelling on the radial side of the wrist and possibly into the hand • Patient will have pain and reduced strength with gripping	• MRA is considered more sensitive than MRI for evaluating the ligaments of the wrist[8]

Palmar Wrist Pain

Ulnocarpal Ligament Sprain

HISTORY	MECHANISM OF INJURY	EVALUATION ESSENTIALS
• Patient reports pain and swelling and difficulty moving the wrist • Patient complains of pain on the ulnar side of the wrist	• Abnormal or forced movement at the wrist • Possibly traumatic due to a fall with wrist extended	• Assess AROM and PROM • Inspect wrist for swelling and palpate wrist for tenderness • Evaluate muscle strength in the wrist

KEY FINDINGS	DIAGNOSTIC EVIDENCE
• Patient will have pain with wrist flexor testing • Patients will likely have swelling on the ulnar side of the wrist and possibly into the hand • Patient will have pain and reduced strength with gripping	• MRA is considered more sensitive than MRI for evaluating the ligaments of the wrist[8]

Dorsal Wrist Pain

Extensor Tendinopathy

HISTORY	MECHANISM OF INJURY	EVALUATION ESSENTIALS
• Patient reports aching and stiffness in wrist and hand • Gradual onset • Patient complains of pain with ADLs as time goes on	• Repetitive or forceful gripping, or use of extensors • Sudden increase in activities involving the hand • Possibly traumatic due to a fall	• Assess AROM and PROM • Inspect and palpate wrist and hand • Evaluate muscle strength in the wrist and hand

KEY FINDINGS	DIAGNOSTIC EVIDENCE
• Patient will have pain with wrist extensor testing • Patients may have pins and needles feeling or numbness in the hand • Patient will have pain with opening the hand and extending the fingers	• Extensor carpi ulnaris is the most common tendon affected • Diagnosis is often by physical examination alone, but MRI and ultrasonography can be used to evaluate integrity of the tendons[8]

Dorsal Wrist Pain

Ganglion Cyst

HISTORY	MECHANISM OF INJURY	EVALUATION ESSENTIALS
• Patient reports a mass on the wrist that is sometimes painful • Appears and disappears quickly and changes size • Pain increases as wrist activity increases	• Idiopathic • Common in individuals between the ages of 15 and 40, and women are more likely to have them than men	• Visual inspection of the posterior wrist • Perform AROM and PROM • Evaluate muscle strength and function

KEY FINDINGS	DIAGNOSTIC EVIDENCE
• There will be a visible lump or mass on the posterior wrist • On palpation may feel soft, rubbery, or very hard • The patient may or may not have pain, it depends upon the size of the cyst and what structures it may put pressure on	• Ultrasound is often the imaging modality of choice, with MRI being used if there are significant neurovascular symptoms[9]

Dorsal Wrist Pain

Lunate Dislocation

HISTORY	MECHANISM OF INJURY	EVALUATION ESSENTIALS
• Acute wrist swelling and pain • Patient may or may not report having numbness or tingling depending upon if the median nerve is affected	• Acute injury • Traumatic, high energy with wrist extended with ulnar deviation	• Assess PROM • Inspect wrist for deformity • Refer and radiograph

KEY FINDINGS	DIAGNOSTIC EVIDENCE
• The patient will have pain over the lunate and the history will indicate trauma • There will be pain and swelling over the lunate area	• Radiographic evidence of lunate dislocation is subtle, with reports of up to 25% of cases being misdiagnosed • MRI is considered more sensitive than plain radiographs[10]

Dorsal Wrist Pain

Radial Nerve Injury (Drop-Wrist Deformity)

HISTORY	MECHANISM OF INJURY	EVALUATION ESSENTIALS
• Patient reports not being able to extend wrist or fingers • Pain is described as sharp and burning	• Direct trauma to the nerve • Compression of the radial nerve	• Assess AROM and PROM • Inspect wrist and hand • Evaluate muscle strength

KEY FINDINGS	DIAGNOSTIC EVIDENCE
• There is paralysis of the extensor muscles such that the wrist and fingers cannot be extended • The patient may have sharp and severe pain	• Compression of the radial nerve can occur at various points throughout the elbow and forearm and symptoms are variable • Electrodiagnostic testing may help confirm diagnosis[7]

Dorsal Wrist Pain

Radiocarpal Ligament Sprain

HISTORY	MECHANISM OF INJURY	EVALUATION ESSENTIALS
• Patient reports pain and swelling and difficulty moving the wrist • Patient complains of pain on the radial side of the wrist posteriorly	• Abnormal or forced movement at the wrist • Possibly traumatic due to a fall with wrist flexed	• Assess AROM and PROM • Inspect wrist for swelling and palpate wrist for tenderness • Evaluate muscle strength in the wrist

KEY FINDINGS	DIAGNOSTIC EVIDENCE
• Patient will have pain with wrist extensor testing • Patients will likely have swelling on the radial side of the wrist and possibly into the hand posteriorly • Patient will have pain when opening the hand and extending the wrist	• MRA is considered more sensitive than MRI for evaluating the ligaments of the wrist[8]

Dorsal Wrist Pain

Ulnocarpal Ligament Sprain

HISTORY

- Patient reports pain and swelling and difficulty moving the wrist
- Patient complains of pain on the ulnar side of the wrist posteriorly

MECHANISM OF INJURY

- Abnormal or forced movement at the wrist
- Possibly traumatic due to a fall with wrist flexed

EVALUATION ESSENTIALS

- Assess AROM and PROM
- Inspect wrist for swelling and palpate wrist for tenderness
- Evaluate muscle strength in the wrist

KEY FINDINGS

- Patient will have pain with wrist extensor testing
- Patients will likely have swelling on the ulnar side of the wrist and possibly into the hand posteriorly
- Patient will have pain with opening the hand and extending the wrist

DIAGNOSTIC EVIDENCE

- MRA is considered more sensitive than MRI for evaluating the ligaments of the wrist[8]

Ulnar Wrist Pain

Triangular Fibrocartilage Complex Injury

HISTORY	MECHANISM OF INJURY	EVALUATION ESSENTIALS
• Patient reports wrist pain clicking and or catching • Pain identified with extension, twist, or rotation of the wrist	• Trauma • Forearm rotation with force loaded through the ulnar portion of the wrist • Forced hyperextension of the wrist (FOOSH) • TFCC pain may be due to degeneration (TFCC has poor blood supply)	• Assess wrist deviation, wrist extension, and/or forearm rotation • Inspect wrist for swelling • TFCC load test • Evaluate muscle strength

KEY FINDINGS	DIAGNOSTIC EVIDENCE
• Swelling may not be much initially • The patient will have pain over the ulnar side of the wrist • Positive TFCC load test with reproduction of pain and symptoms • Is often associated with a sprain of the ulnar collateral ligament, and can exist with a distal radial fracture	• MRA (sensitivity 84%, specificity 95%)[8]

Ulnar Wrist Pain

Ulnar Collateral Ligament Sprain

HISTORY

- Patient reports medial wrist pain
- Pain identified with wrist deviation

MECHANISM OF INJURY

- FOOSH with radial deviation
- Repetitive activity involving rotation or deviation of the wrist

EVALUATION ESSENTIALS

- Perform radial and ulnar deviation
- Assess AROM and PROM
- Inspect medial wrist for swelling
- Evaluate muscle strength about the wrist

KEY FINDINGS

- The patient will have medial wrist pain on palpation
- Patient may have pain with both radial and ulnar deviation
- There will be swelling over the medial side of the wrist

DIAGNOSTIC EVIDENCE

- MRA is considered more sensitive than MRI for evaluating the ligaments of the wrist[8]

Ulnar Wrist Pain

Ulnar Nerve Injury (Benediction or Bishop's Deformity)

HISTORY	MECHANISM OF INJURY	EVALUATION ESSENTIALS
• Patient reports not being able to extend wrist or fingers • Pain is described as sharp and burning	• Direct trauma to the nerve • Compression of the ulnar nerve	• Assess AROM and PROM • Inspect wrist and hand • Evaluate muscle strength

KEY FINDINGS	DIAGNOSTIC EVIDENCE
• There is paralysis of the hypothenar and intrinsic muscles of the fourth and fifth digits • The patient may have sharp and severe pain	• The most common sites of compression are at the cubital tunnel and the Guyon canal in the wrist • Electrodiagnostic testing may be used in conjunction with clinical findings to confirm diagnosis[7]

Radial Wrist Pain

Radial Collateral Ligament Sprain

HISTORY

- Patient reports lateral wrist pain
- Pain identified with wrist deviation

MECHANISM OF INJURY

- FOOSH with ulnar deviation
- Repetitive activity involving rotation or deviation of the wrist

EVALUATION ESSENTIALS

- Perform radial and ulnar deviation
- Assess AROM and PROM
- Inspect lateral wrist for swelling
- Evaluate muscle strength about the wrist

KEY FINDINGS

- The patient will have lateral wrist pain on palpation
- Patient may have pain with both radial and ulnar deviation
- There will be swelling over the lateral side of the wrist

DIAGNOSTIC EVIDENCE

- MRA is considered more sensitive than MRI for evaluating the ligaments of the wrist[8]

Anatomy Map: Wrist and Hand

THUMB

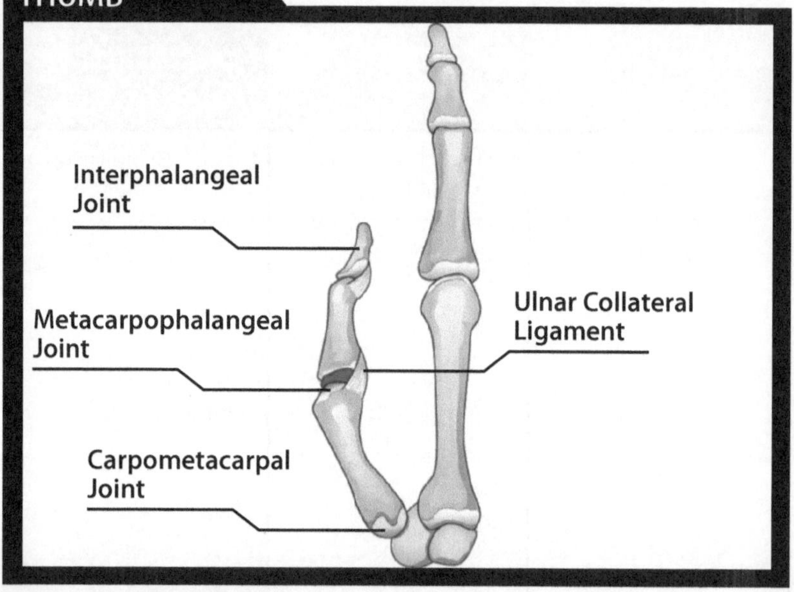

CARPAL TUNNEL

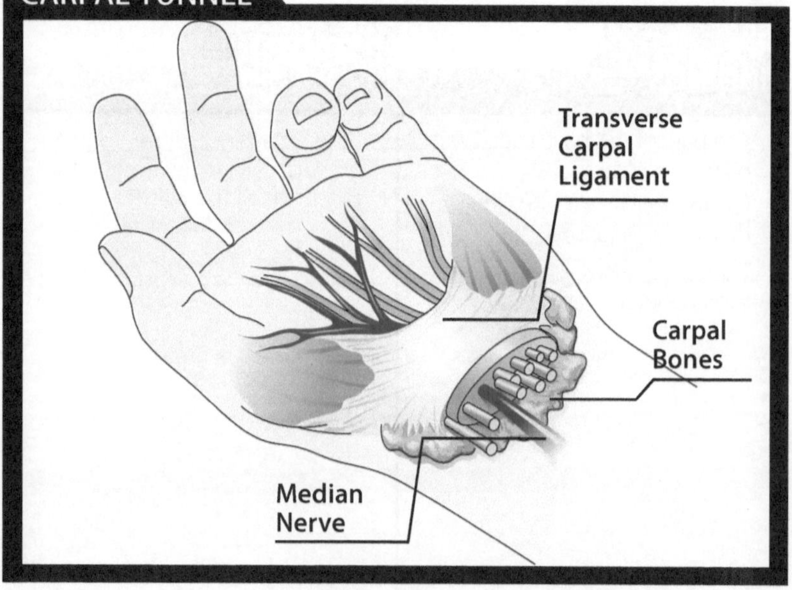

Hand Map: Region/Soft Tissue Differential Diagnosis

PALMAR

Hand/Fingers

- Flexor Tendon Rupture (Jersey Finger)
- Flexor Tendon Sheath Adhesion/ Tenosynovitis (Trigger Finger)
- PIP Palmar Dislocation

Thumb

- IP Joint Capsule Sprain
- MCP Joint Capsule Sprain

DORSAL

Hand/Fingers

- Central Slip Rupture (Boutonniere Deformity)
- DIP Joint Capsule Sprain
- PIP Joint Capsule Sprain
- Extensor Tendon Rupture (Mallet Finger)
- Volar Plate Rupture (Pseudo-Boutonniere Deformity)
- Volar Plate Rupture (Swan-Neck Deformity)

Thumb

- IP Joint Capsule Sprain
- MCP Joint Capsule Sprain
- PIP Dorsal Dislocation
- MCP Dislocation

ULNAR

Hand/Fingers

- Cubital Tunnel Syndrome (Distal Presentation)
- DIP/PIP Ulnar Collateral Ligament Sprain
- Ulnar Nerve Injury (Bishop's Deformity)

Thumb

- MCP Ulnar Collateral Ligament (UCL) Sprain (Gamekeeper's Thumb)

RADIAL

Hand/Fingers

- DIP/PIP Radial Collateral Ligament Sprain

Thumb

- deQuervain's Syndrome

Clinical Assessment of Hand Injuries

Palmar Hand Pain

Flexor Tendon Rupture (Jersey Finger)

HISTORY	MECHANISM OF INJURY	EVALUATION ESSENTIALS
• Pain at the end of the finger • Patient reports trying to grab an opponent's jersey • Patient unable to flex the end of the finger	• Avulsion of the flexor digitorum profundus often accompanies the rupture of the tendon • Forced extension against an actively flexing flexor digitorum profundus • It is most common in the fourth digit	• Assess flexion at each joint in the finger • Inspect distal interphalangeal (DIP) joint for extension deformity • Perform AROM and PROM • Refer for radiograph to assess if an avulsion occured • Evaluate muscle strength

KEY FINDINGS	DIAGNOSTIC EVIDENCE
• The patient's DIP joint is resting in extension and cannot be actively flexed • Patient can still flex at the metacarpal phalangeal (MCP) and proximal interphalangeal (PIP) as the flexor digitorum superficialis is still in tact • There will be pain and swelling to ensue	• Up to 75% of cases occur at the fourth digit • Radiographs may show an avulsion fracture at the distal phalanx[11]

Palmar Hand Pain

Flexor Tendon Sheath Adhesion/Tenosynovitis (Trigger Finger)

HISTORY	MECHANISM OF INJURY	EVALUATION ESSENTIALS
• Patient reports a snap and finger is stuck in flexion • Pain identified with trying to extend finger	• Swelling in the tendons occur and motion is not allowed such that the finger gets stuck in flexion • Thickening of the A1 pulley area • Repetitive movement or non specific overuse • This can occur in one or all fingers including the thumb	• Assess AROM and PROM • Inspect all fingers • Evaluate muscle strength

KEY FINDINGS	DIAGNOSTIC EVIDENCE
• There will be crepitus and painful movement • There is a palpable lump at the base of the flexor tendon sheath and palpable snapping	• Imaging is not usually necessary with trigger finger • To confirm diagnosis, injection of lidocaine into the flexor sheath will relieve pain and allow the finger to be passively or actively extended[12]

Palmar Hand Pain

PIP Palmar Dislocation

HISTORY	MECHANISM OF INJURY	EVALUATION ESSENTIALS
• Patient reports pain and swelling over the PIP • Pain identified at the time of injury and continues	• Twist of a finger while it is semi-flexed	• Assess PROM • Inspect for deformity and palpate • Splint and referral for reduction • Evaluate muscle strength

KEY FINDINGS	DIAGNOSTIC EVIDENCE
• There is an obvious angular or rotational deformity • There is disability with the finger	• Radiographs are often necessary to determine presence of a fracture and stability of the injury[2]

Palmar Hand Pain

Thumb IP Joint Capsule Sprain

HISTORY	MECHANISM OF INJURY	EVALUATION ESSENTIALS
• Patient reports jamming the thumb • Pain identified with moving the thumb or trying to grip	• A hyperextension force in sports with a ball or net • FOOSH with forced thumb abduction (eg, fall while skiing)	• Perform AROM and PROM testing • Assess compression with axial loading and distraction with a P/A glide • Inspect thumb for swelling or ecchymosis and pain • Evaluate muscle strength

KEY FINDINGS	DIAGNOSTIC EVIDENCE
• The patient will have pain on the anterior aspect of the IP joint • Patient will likely have laxity with P/A glide • The patient will have pain and a history to go along with findings	• No diagnostic evidence available

Palmar Hand Pain

Thumb MCP Joint Capsule Sprain

HISTORY	MECHANISM OF INJURY	EVALUATION ESSENTIALS
• Patient reports jamming the thumb • Pain identified with moving the thumb or trying to grip	• A hyperextension force in sports with a ball or net • FOOSH with forced thumb abduction (eg, fall while skiing)	• Perform AROM and PROM testing • Assess compression with axial loading and distraction with a P/A glide • Inspect thumb for swelling or ecchymosis and pain • Evaluate muscle strength

KEY FINDINGS	DIAGNOSTIC EVIDENCE
• The patient will have pain on the anterior aspect of the MCP joint • Patient will likely have laxity with P/A glide • The patient will have pain and a history to go along with findings	• No diagnostic evidenc available

Dorsal Hand Pain

Central Slip Rupture (Boutonniere Deformity)

HISTORY	MECHANISM OF INJURY	EVALUATION ESSENTIALS
• Patient reports inability to extend the DIP joint • Trauma to finger in history • Pain is severe and identified with moving the finger	• Rupture of the extensor tendon dorsal to the middle phalanx • Trauma to the tip of the finger forcing DIP into extension and the PIP into flexion	• Perform PROM of joints at the finger • Assess deformity of the DIP and PIP joints • Inspect finger for swelling and point tenderness • Evaluate muscle strength

KEY FINDINGS	DIAGNOSTIC EVIDENCE
• The patient will be in severe pain with swelling and point tenderness • The patient will not be able to extend the DIP joint • The patient will have an obvious deformity	• Radiographs and MRI may be used to determine the need for surgical intervention[11]

Dorsal Hand Pain

DIP Joint Capsule Sprain

HISTORY	MECHANISM OF INJURY	EVALUATION ESSENTIALS
• Patient reports jamming the finger • Pain identified with moving the finger or trying to grip	• A hyperflexion force in sports with a ball or net • Falling on outstretched arm with finger flexed	• Perform AROM and PROM testing • Assess compression with axial loading and distraction with a A/P glide • Inspect finger for swelling or ecchymosis and pain • Evaluate muscle strength

KEY FINDINGS	DIAGNOSTIC EVIDENCE
• The patient will have pain on the posterior aspect of the DIP joint • Patient will likely have laxity with A/P glide • The patient will have pain and a history to go along with findings	• Radiographs may be warranted to rule out an avulsion fracture[13]

Dorsal Hand Pain

PIP Joint Capsule Sprain

HISTORY	MECHANISM OF INJURY	EVALUATION ESSENTIALS
• Patient reports jamming the finger • Pain identified with moving the finger or trying to grip	• A hyperflexion force in sports with a ball or net • Falling on outstretched arm with finger flexed • Forced varus or valgus stress	• Perform AROM and PROM testing • Assess compression with axial loading and distraction with a A/P glide • Inspect finger for swelling or ecchymosis and pain • Evaluate muscle strength

KEY FINDINGS	DIAGNOSTIC EVIDENCE
• The patient will have pain on the posterior aspect of the PIP joint • Patient will likely have laxity with A/P glide • The patient will have pain and a history to go along with findings	• Radiographs may be warranted to rule out an avulsion fracture[13]

Dorsal Hand Pain

Extensor Tendon Rupture (Mallet Finger)

HISTORY	MECHANISM OF INJURY	EVALUATION ESSENTIALS
• Patient reports pain at the DIP joint • Patient complains of not being able to extend the finger • May report being hit with a ball on end of the finger	• When an extended finger is abruptly forced into flexion at the DIP joint • Laceration to the distal dorsal finger • A DIP hyperextension resulting in a fracture to the base of the distal phalanx and trauma to the distal finger	• Assess all joints at the finger • Perform PROM testing • Referral and radiograph may be necessary • Evaluate muscle strength

KEY FINDINGS	DIAGNOSTIC EVIDENCE
• The patient will not be able to extend the finger • If there is an avulsion of bone you can palpate it	• Radiographs or CT can identify avulsion fractures at the distal phalanx[11]

Dorsal Hand Pain

Volar Plate Rupture (Pseudo-Boutonniere Deformity)

HISTORY

- Patient reports a hyperextension injury
- Pain identified with trying to move the finger

MECHANISM OF INJURY

- Severe hyperextension force
- An avulsion of the volar plate from the proximal phalanx

EVALUATION ESSENTIALS

- Assess the joints of the finger
- Inspect for deformity
- Perform PROM tests
- Referral and radiograph necessary
- Evaluate muscle strength

KEY FINDINGS

- The patient will have pain and swelling over the volar side of the PIP joint
- The difference between this and Swan-Neck deformity is the avulsion of the volar plate and this must be referred

DIAGNOSTIC EVIDENCE

- Radiographs are often necessary to determine presence of a fracture and stability of the injury[2]

Dorsal Hand Pain

Volar Plate Rupture (Swan-Neck Deformity)

HISTORY	MECHANISM OF INJURY	EVALUATION ESSENTIALS
• Patient reports a hyperextension injury • Pain identified with trying to move the finger	• Severe hyperextension force • A distal tear of the volar plate from the middle phalanx	• Assess the joints of the finger • Inspect for deformity • Perform PROM tests • Evaluate muscle strength

KEY FINDINGS	DIAGNOSTIC EVIDENCE
• The patient will have pain and swelling over the volar side of the PIP joint • The PIP can be passively extended in comparison to the other PIP joints	• Radiographs are often necessary to determine presence of a fracture and stability of the injury[2]

Dorsal Hand Pain

Thumb IP Joint Capsule Sprain

HISTORY

- Patient reports jamming the thumb
- Pain identified with moving the thumb or trying to grip

MECHANISM OF INJURY

- A hyperflexion force in sports with a ball or net
- Falling on outstretched arm with thumb flexed
- Forced varus and valgus stress

EVALUATION ESSENTIALS

- Perform AROM and PROM testing
- Assess compression with axial loading, and distraction with a A/P glide
- Inspect thumb for swelling or ecchymosis and pain
- Evaluate muscle strength

KEY FINDINGS

- The patient will have pain on the posterior aspect of the IP joint
- Patient will likely have laxity with A/P glide
- The patient will have pain and a history to go along with findings

DIAGNOSTIC EVIDENCE

- Radiographs may be warranted to rule out an avulsion fracture[13]

Dorsal Hand Pain

Thumb MCP Joint Capsule Sprain

HISTORY	MECHANISM OF INJURY	EVALUATION ESSENTIALS
• Patient reports jamming the thumb • Pain identified with moving the thumb or trying to grip	• A hyperflexion force in sports with a ball or net • Falling on outstretched arm with thumb flexed • Forced varus and valgus stress	• Perform AROM and PROM testing • Assess compression with axial loading and distraction with a A/P glide • Inspect thumb for swelling or ecchymosis and pain • Evaluate muscle strength

KEY FINDINGS	DIAGNOSTIC EVIDENCE
• The patient will have pain on the posterior aspect of the MCP joint • Patient will likely have laxity with A/P glide • The patient will have pain and a history to go along with findings	• No diagnostic evidence available

Dorsal Hand Pain

Thumb PIP Dorsal Dislocation

HISTORY	MECHANISM OF INJURY	EVALUATION ESSENTIALS
• Patient reports pain and swelling over the PIP • Pain identified at the time of injury and continues	• Hyperextension that produces disruption of the volar plate at the middle phalanx • Common dislocation	• Assess PROM • Inspect for deformity and palpate • Splint and referral for reduction • Evaluate muscle strength

KEY FINDINGS	DIAGNOSTIC EVIDENCE
• There is an obvious avulsion deformity • There is disability with the finger	• Radiographs are often necessary to determine presence of a fracture and stability of the injury[2]

Dorsal Hand Pain

Thumb MCP Dislocation

HISTORY	MECHANISM OF INJURY	EVALUATION ESSENTIALS
• Patient reports pain and swelling and stiffness over the MCP • Pain identified at the time of injury and continues	• Twisting or shear force	• Assess PROM • Inspect for deformity and palpate • Splint and referral for reduction • Evaluate muscle strength

KEY FINDINGS	DIAGNOSTIC EVIDENCE
• There is an obvious avulsion deformity • The distal phalanx is dorsally angulated at 60 to 90 degrees • There is disability with the finger	• Radiographs can determine the presence of a fracture and the stability of the injury[2]

Ulnar Hand Pain

Cubital Tunnel Syndrome (Distal Presentation)

HISTORY	MECHANISM OF INJURY	EVALUATION ESSENTIALS
• Patient complains of medial elbow pain that radiates into the ulnar aspect of the hand • Patient may experience burning and tingling the fourth and fifth fingers • May wake with tingling in the last two fingers • Pain identified with hyperflexion	• Pronounced cubitus valgus developing friction or subluxing of ulnar nerve • Ulnar nerve can become impinged with repetitive flexion activity • Traction injury from a valgus force • Irregularities in the tunnel	• Assess throwing mechanics if appropriate • Identify elbow posture in anatomical postion • Tinel's test • Perform AROM and PROM testing • Evaluate muscle strength

KEY FINDINGS	DIAGNOSTIC EVIDENCE
• While technically an elbow condition, patients frequently feel symptoms in the ulnar side of the hand • The patient will likely present with a valgus deformity of the elbow • Patient will experience a popping with flexion and extension of the elbow • The patient will experience burning and or tingling in the fourth and fifth fingers • The patient may note a change in sensation	• History and physical examination alone are often enough to diagnose this syndrome, but electrodiagnostic testing may be used for confirmation[14]

Ulnar Hand Pain

DIP/PIP Ulnar Collateral Ligament Sprain

HISTORY	MECHANISM OF INJURY	EVALUATION ESSENTIALS
• Patient reports jamming their finger • Patient reports pain and swelling of the finger • Pain identified with moving finger or gripping	• An axial force that places valgus stress at the joint	• Valgus stress testing at the PIP joint • Assess AROM and PROM • Inspect joint and palpate • Evaluate muscle strength

KEY FINDINGS	DIAGNOSTIC EVIDENCE
• The patient will have laxity and pain with valgus testing • Must refer if there is no end point with valgus testing • The patient will have severe tenderness over the ulnar collateral ligament	• No diagnostic evidence available

Ulnar Hand Pain

Ulnar Nerve Injury (Bishop's Deformity)

HISTORY	MECHANISM OF INJURY	EVALUATION ESSENTIALS
• Patient reports not being able to extend wrist or fingers • Pain is described as sharp and burning	• Direct trauma to the nerve • Compression of the ulnar nerve	• Assess AROM and PROM • Inspect wrist and hand • Evaluate muscle strength

KEY FINDINGS	DIAGNOSTIC EVIDENCE
• There is paralysis of the hypothenar and intrinsic muscles of the fourth and fifth digits • The patient may have sharp and severe pain	• Electrodiagnostic testing (sensitivity 37% to 86%, specificity 95%)[15]

Ulnar Hand Pain

MCP Ulnar Collateral Ligament Sprain (Gamekeeper's Thumb)

HISTORY	MECHANISM OF INJURY	EVALUATION ESSENTIALS
• Patient reports pain at the MCP joint • Pain identifies weakness and painful when trying to pinch • Patient will describe a logical mechanism of injury	• Forceful abduction of the proximal phalanx sometimes combined with hyperextension • Fall while skiing or forceful abduction from ski pole	• Assess MCP joint • Inspect for swelling and point tenderness • Valgus stress testing • Assess AROM and PROM • Evaluate muscle strength

KEY FINDINGS	DIAGNOSTIC EVIDENCE
• There is tenderness and swelling over the medial thumb • Positive valgus stress testing; refer immediately if no end point	• Radiographs can identify avulsion fractures at the ulnar aspect of the base of the first metacarpal[11]

Radial Hand Pain

DIP/PIP Radial Collateral Ligament Sprain

HISTORY	MECHANISM OF INJURY	EVALUATION ESSENTIALS
• Patient reports jamming his or her finger • Patient reports pain and swelling of the finger • Pain identified with moving finger or gripping	• An axial force that places varus stress at the joint	• Valgus stress testing at the IP joint • Assess AROM and PROM • Inspect joint and palpate • Evaluate muscle strength

KEY FINDINGS	DIAGNOSTIC EVIDENCE
• The patient will have laxity and pain with varus testing • Must refer if there is no end point with varus testing • The patient will have severe tenderness over the radial collateral ligament	• No diagnostic evidence available

Radial Hand Pain

deQuervain's Syndrome

HISTORY	MECHANISM OF INJURY	EVALUATION ESSENTIALS
• Patient reports snapping that is painful • Patient complains of catching during movement of the thumb • Pain identified as aching and radiates to thumb and or forearm	• Tenosynovitis that is stenosing at the thumb • Narrowing tunnel as a result of inflammation of tendons • Wrist motion is a source of pain due to the way the tendons move through the narrow tunnel	• Assess AROM and PROM • Inspect for crepitus and palpate for pain • Finkelstein's test • Evaluate muscle strength

KEY FINDINGS	DIAGNOSTIC EVIDENCE
• There is point tenderness and weakness with thumb extension and abduction • There is painful snapping and catching with motion	• Diagnosis is usually based on clinical examination, but MRI and ultrasound can aid in identifying inflammation of tendons • Sensitivity and specificity of Finkelstein's test are unknown[16]

Paper Patient: Revisited

You should have been able to rule out several conditions secondary to knowing what structures are at the thumb and hand. Your differential should have been carpal tunnel syndrome versus deQuervain's syndrome.

Learning Activities: Practice Case

Use the blank templates provided in the Appendices to write out a differential diagnosis map and clinical findings overview for the case provided below. When working with paper patients, it is tempting to try to jump to "the answer" and come to a diagnosis. However, the visual learning approach to differential diagnosis is designed to help you consider all the possibilities for the information provided. Good luck.

Paper Patient: Thumb Pain in a Recreational Basketball Player

History

Ricardo is a 22-year-old college student who injured his right thumb while playing basketball 5 days ago. He states that he reached out to block and pass and "jammed" his thumb. He states that he still has pain with motion. He expected the pain to be gone by now. He reports that he used ice on the thumb for a day or so and has taken ibuprofen as needed. He states that it still looks and feels swollen and is painful (4/10). Ricardo is right hand dominant. He also is a member of the baseball team at his school (outfield and pitcher). He has been avoiding these activities since the time of his injury. Ricardo indicates that the interphalangeal joint is the site of his pain.

Physical Exam

The physical exam reveals that AROM of the first IP and MCP are WNL. Movement of the first IP joint is painful (5/10). PROM is WNL with normal end feel and is also painful (4/10). Varus and valgus stress tests of the IP are negative. A ligamentous exam of the MCP joint is normal and there is no bony tenderness. The patient has normal sensation and capillary refill.

References

1. Rettig AC. Athletic injuries of the wrist and hand. Part I: Traumatic injuries of the wrist. *Am J Sports Med.* 2003;31:1038–1048.
2. Rettig AC. Athletic injuries of the wrist and hand. Part II: Overuse injuries of the wrist and traumatic injuries to the hand. *Am J Sports Med.* 2004;32(1):262-273.
3. Swenson DM, Yard EE, Collins CL, et al. Epidemiology of US high school sports-related fractures, 2005–2009. *Clin J Sport Med.* 2010;20:293-299.
4. Rettig AC, Patel DV. Epidemiology of elbow, forearm, and wrist injuries in the athlete. *Clin Sports Med.* 1995;14:289 -297.
5. Logan AJ. Acute hand and wrist injuries in experienced rock climbers. *Br J Sports Med.* 2004;38(5):545-548.
6. Fufa DT, Goldfarb CA. Sports injuries of the wrist. *Curr Rev Musculoskelet Med.* 2013;6(1):35-40.
7. Popinchalk SP, Schaffer AA. Physical examination of upper extremity compressive neuropathies. *Orthop Clin North Am.* 2012;43(4):417-430.
8. Bancroft LW. Wrist injuries: A comparison between high- and low-impact sports. *Radiol Clin North Am.* 2013;51(2):299-311.
9. Freire V, Guérini H, Campagna R, et al. Imaging of hand and wrist cysts: A clinical approach. *AJR Am J Roentgenol.* 2012;199(5):W618-628.
10. Jones DB Jr, Kakar S. Perilunate dislocations and fracture dislocations. *J Hand Surg Am.* 2012;37(10):2168-2173.
11. Peterson JJ, Bancroft LW. Injuries of the fingers and thumb in the athlete. *Clin Sports Med.* 2006;25(3):527-542.
12. Makkouk AH, Oetgen ME, Swigart CR, Dodds SD. Trigger finger: Etiology, evaluation, and treatment. *Curr Rev Musculoskelet Med.* 2008;1(2):92-96.
13. Leggit JC, Meko CJ. Acute finger injuries: Part I. Tendons and ligaments. *Am Fam Physician.* 2006;73(5):810-816.
14. Kroonen LT. Cubital tunnel syndrome. *Orthop Clin North Am.* 2012;43(4):475-486.
15. Werner RA. Electrodiagnostic evaluation of carpal tunnel syndrome and ulnar neuropathies. *PMR.* 2013;5(5 Suppl):S14-21.
16. Batteson R, Hammond A, Burke F, Sinha S. The de Quervain's screening tool: Validity and reliability of a measure to support clinical diagnosis and management. *Musculoskeletal Care.* 2008;6(3):168-180.

10

The Head and Face

The popularity of sport and recreational physical activity in the United States is undeniable. Each year nearly 40 million children and over 150 million adults participate in organized sport and physical activities. Many of these sports carry an increased risk of sustaining a head injury.[1] An estimated 1.6 to 3.8 million concussions occur in sports and recreational activities annually in the United States, many of whom do not obtain immediate medical attention.[2,3] Because of the greater number of male participants in sports studied by researchers, the total number of reported concussions is larger for males than females for all sports combined. However, the relationship of concussion risk and sex varies among sports. Studies indicated that the concussion risk is greater for female athletes participating in soccer or basketball.[4,5] Traumatic brain injuries (TBI) occur in an estimated 1.7 million people and account for over 1.3 million emergency room visits and 275,000 hospitalizations annually.[6] The cost of these injuries is significant with an estimated $60 billion in direct and indirect expenses estimated annually.[7] These estimates do not account for individuals suffering from mild to moderate TBI and do not seek medical care.

There has been an elevated awareness of concussion assessment, management, and treatment in recent years. Despite this increased awareness, the diagnosis of concussion and some aspects of its management can present a challenge for the sports medicine team. Clinicians must be well versed in current evaluation techniques, sideline assessment tools, and symptoms

Winterstein AP, Clark SV. *The Athletic Trainer's Guide to Differential Diagnosis (pp 321–356).*

checklist instruments when managing possible brain trauma. In addition clinicians must keep abreast of the most recent concussion guidelines[8] and positions statements[9] guiding clinical practice.

In addition to the emphasis on concussion, injuries to the face and related structures present a unique challenge for the athletic trainer. Clinicians must be fully aware of the wide range of injuries that can occur to the face and the related structures (eg, eye, nose, ear) while at the same time never forgetting that trauma to the brain is always a possibility. The same injury mechanism that may result in an injury to the face may very well have caused an underlying concussive force to the brain. The differential diagnosis map for this chapter is divided by structures and not regions; and separate information is provided on traumatic brain injury. Students in training will do well to remember not to be misled by the obvious injury and always remember to fully evaluate the brain when dealing with injuries to the head and face.

Paper Patient: Head Injury in an Ice Hockey Player

History

Casey is an 18-year-old hockey player who was checked into the boards at full speed and fell to the ice hitting his head. The on ice evaluation found him to be unconscious initially for about 20-30 seconds according to the referee. He comes to consciousness quickly once you call out his name.

Physical Exam

Your physical exam on the ice reveals no tenderness over the cervical spine. He does not have retro- or anterograde amnesia. The patient reports a mild headache. His pupils are equal and reactive to light. His cranial nerve assessment was also negative.

After ten minutes symptoms begin to worsen with increased dizziness, nausea, sleepiness, and severe headache

Clinical Decisions

Using the information from your clinical exam you will need to ask yourself some questions to guide your clinical decision making:

- What is your differential diagnosis?
- What key findings do you see to help guide your differential?

- What are the possible injuries associated with head injury?

Start with a review of the anatomy maps and a thorough consideration of the possible injuries and conditions that are common to the head and face. Use the differential diagnosis maps to guide your thought process and organize the possibilities. The organized synthesis of this information is the essence of clinical decision making. We will revisit this case at the end of the chapter.

Anatomy Map: Head

ANTERIOR

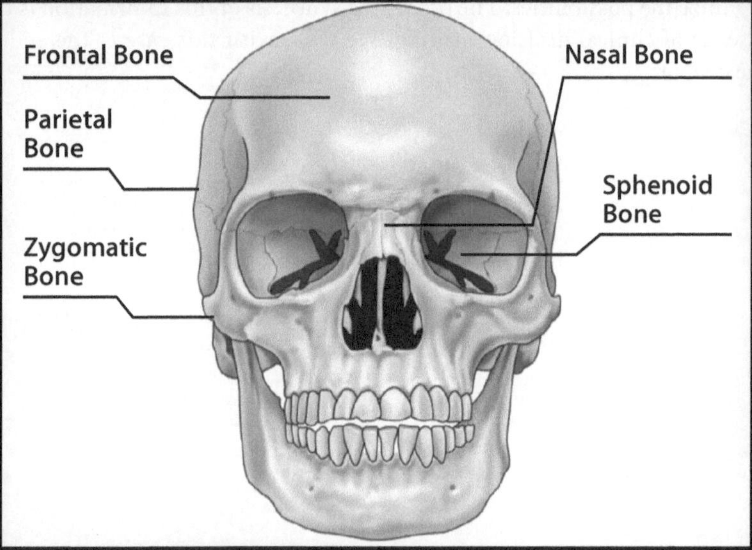

POSTERIOR

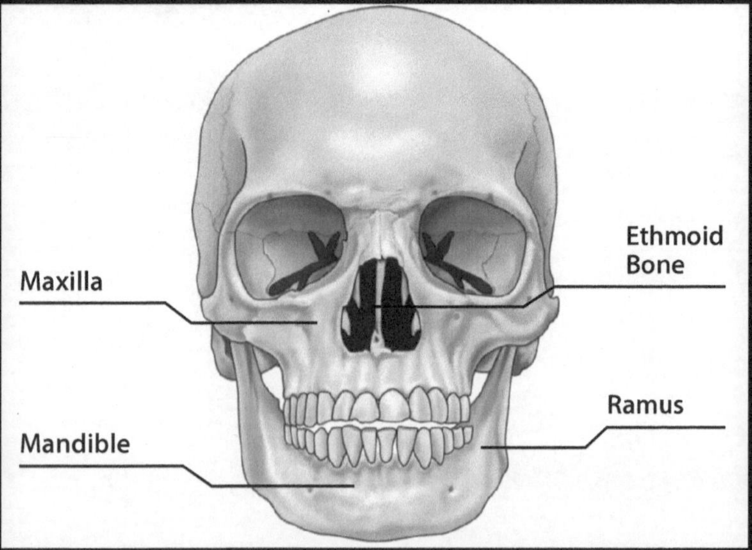

Anatomy Map: Head

EAR

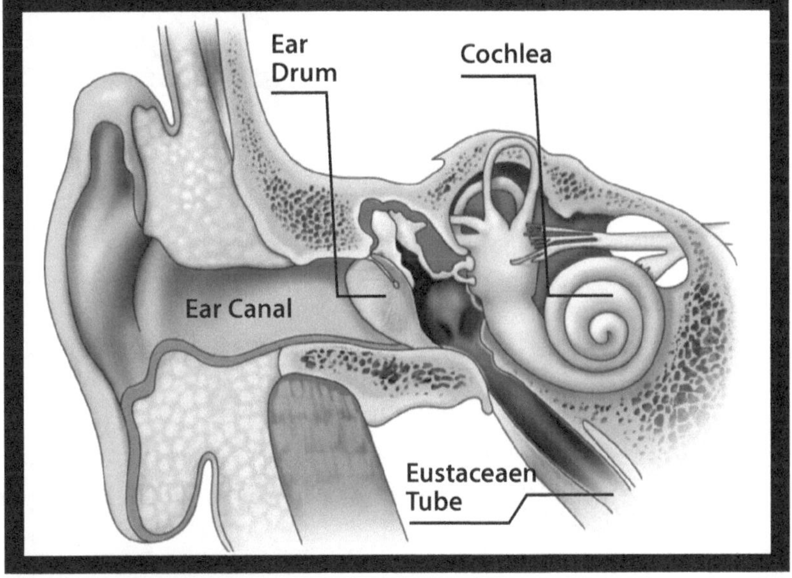

EYE

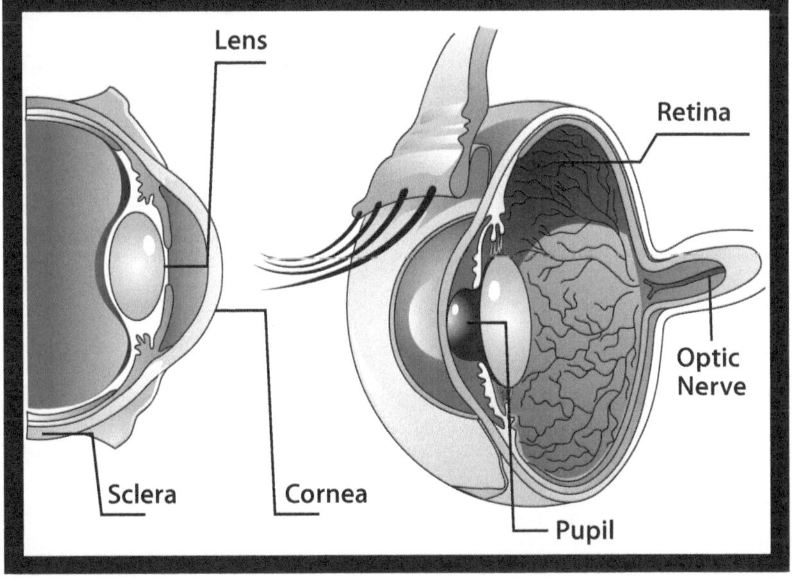

Mild Traumatic Brain Injury/Concussion

Concussion

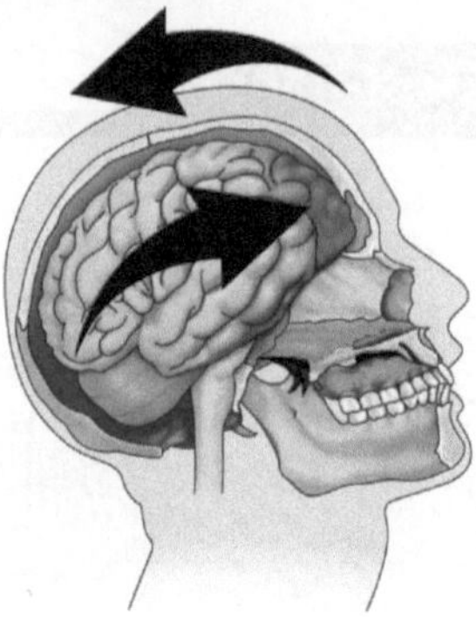

- A concussion is a brain injury and is defined as a complex pathophysiological process affecting the brain, induced by biomechanical forces. Several common features of a concussive head injury are as follows.
    - Concussion may be caused either by a direct blow to the head, face, neck or elsewhere on the body with an "impulsive" force transmitted to the head.
    - Concussion typically results in the rapid onset of short-lived impairment of neurological function that resolves spontaneously. However, in some cases, symptoms and signs may evolve over a number of minutes to hours.
    - Concussion may result in neuropathological changes, but the acute clinical symptoms largely reflect a functional disturbance rather than a structural injury.
    - Concussion results in a graded set of clinical symptoms that may or may not involve loss of consciousness. Resolution of the clinical and cognitive symptoms typically follows a sequential course. However, it is important to note that in some cases symptoms may be prolonged.

Adapted from McCrory P, et al. "Consensus statement on concussion in sport: the 4th International Conference on Concussion in Sport held in Zurich, November 2012." *BJSM* 47.5 (2013): 250-258.

Brain Injury

Traumatic and Mild Traumatic Brain Injury

TERMS AND DEFINITIONS

- **Traumatic Brain Injury**
  - Traumatic brain injury (TBI) is also known as intracranial injury, occurs when an external force traumatically injures the brain. TBI is usually classified based on severity or mechanism (closed or penetrating head injury).
- **Mild Traumatic Brain Injury**
  - Mild traumatic brain injury (mTBI) and concussion are often used interchangeably; mTBI is a subset of TBI (see concussion definition box on page 326).
- **Subdural Hematoma**
  - A subdural hematoma forms when blood (usually venous) gathers within the outermost meningeal layer, between the dura mater and the arachnoid mater of the brain. This buildup of blood can cause an increase in intracranial pressure leading to further brain injury.
  - Three types (acute, subacute, and chronic) may develop.
- **Epidural Hematoma**
  - An epidural hematoma occurs when blood accumulates between the skull and the dura mater, the thick membrane covering the brain.
  - They typically occur when a skull fracture tears an underlying blood vessel (arterial).
  - Rapid diagnosis and surgical intervention are needed to prevent death.

Brain Injury

EVALUATION

- The diagnosis of acute concussion usually involves the assessment of a range of domains including clinical symptoms, physical signs, cognitive impairment, neurobehavioral features, and sleep disturbance. A detailed concussion history is an important part of the evaluation both in the injured athlete and when conducting a preparticipation examination.
- Clinicians are encouraged to use a symptom checklist like the Sport Concussion Assessment Tool (SCAT3) to aide in their assessment.
- The suspected diagnosis of concussion can include one or more of the following clinical domains:
  - **Symptoms:** somatic (eg, headache), cognitive (eg, feeling like in a fog) and/or emotional symptoms (eg, lability)
  - **Physical signs** (eg, loss of consciousness (LOC), amnesia)
  - **Behavioral changes** (eg, irritability)
  - **Cognitive impairment** (eg, slowed reaction times)
  - **Sleep disturbance** (eg, insomnia)
- If any one or more of these components are present, a concussion should be suspected and the appropriate management strategy instituted.

Adapted from McCrory P, et al. "Consensus statement on concussion in sport: the 4th International Conference on Concussion in Sport held in Zurich, November 2012." *BJSM* 47.5 (2013): 250-258.

Brain Injury

Concussion/Mild Traumatic Brain Injury

HISTORY	MECHANISM OF INJURY	EVALUATION ESSENTIALS
• Patient may report blow to the head or violent movement of the head • May describe history of headache, nausea, motor imbalance, and emotional changes • Amnesia may make history difficult	• A direct blow to the head when the athlete's head is moving, resulting in deceleration of the brain • A direct blow to the head by another moving object • Rapid shaking or rotational movement causing intracranial movement of the brain	• Use checklist (eg, SCAT3) • Assess cranial nerves • Inspect for other injury/clear the neck with history and palpation • Assess retrograde and anterograde amnesia • Evaluate balance, motor function, coordination, and cognitive function

KEY FINDINGS	DIAGNOSTIC EVIDENCE
• The patient may have any one or many concussion symptoms such as nausea, headache, photophobia, neck pain, difficulty balancing, antegrade or retrograde amnesia, and any one or several positive cranial nerve tests that are positive. • Refer to box on Brain Injury: Evaluation on page 328 for further details.	• The majority (80% to 90%) of concussions resolve in a short (7 to 10 day) period, although the recovery time frame may be longer in children and adolescents[10] • Persistent symptoms (> 10 days) are generally reported in 10% to 15% of concussions. In general, symptoms are not specific to concussion and it is important to consider other pathologies.[8]

Brain Injury

Epidural Hematoma

HISTORY	MECHANISM OF INJURY	EVALUATION ESSENTIALS
• Patient presents with a blow to the head • Acute onset	• A blow to the head or skull fracture causing an arterial bleed • Because of the arterial blood pressure, blood accumulation and creation of the hematoma occur quickly a few minutes to a few hours	• Assess the patient's cranial nerves • Inspect site of the blow to the head • Evaluate cognition and balance • Refer for CT scan

KEY FINDINGS	DIAGNOSTIC EVIDENCE
• May be lucid for a short time, and then the symptoms return and worsen rapidly to include dizziness, nausea, dilation of one pupil usually on the same side as the injury, and sleepiness • Later stages will present with deteriorating consciousness, neck rigidity, depression of pulse, and respiration as well as convulsions; this is life threatening	• CT scans are the imaging modality of choice for epidural hematomas • Up to 90% of patients with epidural hematomas have an associated skull fracture[11]

Brain Injury

Subdural Hematoma

HISTORY

- Patient presents after receiving a blow to the head
- Acute onset

MECHANISM OF INJURY

- A blow to the head causing a venous bleed
- Occurs more frequently than epidural hematomas and leading cause of death in athletes

EVALUATION ESSENTIALS

- Assess cranial nerves
- Inspect site of the blow to the head
- Evaluate cognition and balance
- Refer for CT scan

KEY FINDINGS

- The patient most likely will not have had a loss of consciousness. Symptoms include dizziness, nausea, and sleepiness. In a complicated subdural hematoma the patient may be unconscious and have dilation of one pupil, usually on the same side as the injury
- This is life threatening

DIAGNOSTIC EVIDENCE

- CT scan is the imaging modality of choice for subdural hematomas
- MRI may be indicated for more diffuse injuries[11]

Brain Injury

Post-Concussive Syndrome

OVERVIEW

- Commonly reported symptoms of concussion include headache, nausea, dizziness and balance problems, blurred vision, confusion, memory disturbance, mental "fogginess," and fatigue.
- The literature has shown that the majority of concussions or mTBI in adults resolve within 10 days of injury. Concussions that fall outside of the expected window of recovery (eg, > 10 days) are sometimes called a "difficult concussion."
- The incidence of prolonged clinical recovery following concussion varies.
- Common persistent symptoms include headache, depression, difficulty concentrating, fatigue or low energy, difficulty sleeping or feeling not quite right, in a fog, or slowed down.
- These symptoms may be reported in healthy athletic populations following concussion and in patients with other injuries, illnesses or neuropsychiatric conditions.
- Cases where clinical recovery falls outside the expected window (ie, 10 days) should be managed in a multidisciplinary manner by providers with sports concussion experience.

Adapted from Makdissi M, Cantu R, Johnston K, McCrory P, Meeuwisse W. The difficult concussion patient: what is the best approach to investigation and management of persistent (>10 days) Postconcussive symptoms? *Br J Sports Med.* 2013;47(5):308-313.

Head/Face Map: Region/Soft Tissue Differential Diagnosis

EYE

- Anisocoria
- Conjunctivitis
- Corneal Abrasion
- Corneal Laceration
- Detached Retina
- Hyphema
- Iritis
- Orbital Hematoma
- Ruptured Globe
- Stye and Blepharitis
- Subconjunctival Hematoma

EAR

- Auricular Hematoma (Cauliflower Ear)
- Otitis Externa (Swimmer's Ear)
- Otitis Media
- Tympanic Membrane Rupture

NOSE

- Deviated Septum
- Epistaxis

MOUTH/JAW

- Mandibular Luxation
- Temporomandibular Joint (TMJ) Dysfunction
- Tooth Luxations
- Trigeminal Neuralgia

Head/Face

Injuries to Bone

COMMON FRACTURES

- LeFort fractures
- Mandibular fracture
- Maxillary fracture
- Nasal fracture
- Orbital blow-out fracture
- Skull fractures
- Tooth fractures
- Zygoma fracture

Note: High velocity forces that can cause fractures to the skull and face may result in concomitant injuries to the brain. Patients should be evaluated with care and referred for a thorough evaluation to assess both the potential fracture and the underlying possibility of concussion.

Clinical Assessment of Injuries to the Head and Face

Eye

Anisocoria

HISTORY	MECHANISM OF INJURY	EVALUATION ESSENTIALS
• Patient reports that his or her pupils are different size • Patient may experience droopiness of the eye • Patient may complain of difficulty focusing on objects that are near in their field of view	• May be physiologic (approximately 20% of population) and vary day to day with the difference in pupil size between the 2 eyes not to exceed 1 mm • May be due to an underlying medical condition • If pupil is abnormally large, the mechanism can be from trauma or possibly from cranial nerve involvement • If the pupil is abnormally small, it is usually due to inflammation or trauma	• Assess pupil size • Pupil may be sluggish to react to light • Patient may have diminished deep tendon reflexes • Referral to physician is necessary for a full and thorough eye exam

KEY FINDINGS	DIAGNOSTIC EVIDENCE
• There is a difference in pupil size • History and exam will determine whether it is a physiologic or medically based issue	• If anisocoria is present following head trauma, patient should be transported to an emergency department to determine if there is intracranial bleeding or fractures via CT and MRI[12]

Eye

Conjunctivitis

HISTORY	MECHANISM OF INJURY	EVALUATION ESSENTIALS
• Patient reports eyelids crusted shut • Patient complains of swollen eyes • Eye or eyes are itchy and may burn	• Allergens • Bacterial • May be associated with cold or other upper respiratory issue	• Assess for discharge from the eye • Inspect conjunctiva • Evaluate patient for other symptoms and thorough health history

KEY FINDINGS	DIAGNOSTIC EVIDENCE
• The patient will have redness, itchiness, and burning in the eyes • There will be discharge from the eye and crusted eyes in the morning • History will be evident as to the cause of conjunctivitis such as allergens and upper respiratory problems	• No diagnostic evidence available

Eye

Corneal Abrasion

HISTORY	MECHANISM OF INJURY	EVALUATION ESSENTIALS
• Patient reports that the eye is watering and he or she has photophobia • Acute onset • Pain identified with opening and closing the eye	• A foreign body is in the eye and patient rubs his or her eye causing an abrasion of the cornea	• Assess cornea for abrasion by using fluorescein stain and black light • Inspect eye for foreign body • Gently lift upper lid over lower lid while patient looks down to induce tears

KEY FINDINGS	DIAGNOSTIC EVIDENCE
• The patient will complain of a scratching feeling in the eye • The eye will be watery, and the patient will have sensitivity to light • Under the black light, you will see a scratch or abrasion	• Vision loss of more than 20/40 requires referral to an opthamologist to rule out more severe injury[13]

Eye

Detached Retina

HISTORY	MECHANISM OF INJURY	EVALUATION ESSENTIALS
• Patient reports specks floating in the eye, flashes of light, or blurred vision	• Blow to the eye • Detachment is not painful • Retinal detachment is common among athletes who have myopia	• Assess patient's vision • Inspect eye • Referral to physician is necessary immediately to determine if surgery is necessary

KEY FINDINGS	DIAGNOSTIC EVIDENCE
• The patient will have a change in vision • The history will indicate blow to the eye and symptoms of specks floating in the eye, flashing of light or blurred vision will be present	• No diagnostic evidence available

Eye

Hyphema

HISTORY	MECHANISM OF INJURY	EVALUATION ESSENTIALS
• Patient reports that his or her vision is partially or completely blocked • Acute onset	• Blunt blow to the anterior aspect of the eye • It is usually from a ball and the patient is not wearing protective eyewear	• Assess for reddish tinge in the anterior chamber of the eye within the first 2 hours • Inspect eye for blood settling inferiorly or filling the entire chamber • Must refer to MD for thorough eye exam to avoid serious problem with lens, choroids, or retina

KEY FINDINGS	DIAGNOSTIC EVIDENCE
• The eye will start with reddish tinge and when blood settles it may turn pea green color filling the inferior and possibly entire chamber	• No diagnostic evidence available

Eye

Iritis

HISTORY	MECHANISM OF INJURY	EVALUATION ESSENTIALS
• Patient reports reddened eye, small or funny shaped pupil, blurred vision • Typically an acute onset affecting one eye • Pain identified with exposure to bright light • Patient may have pain in the eye or eyebrow region and headache	• Trauma to the eye • Secondary to other diseases such as ankylosing spondylitis, Reiter syndrome, sarcoidosis, inflammatory bowel disease, and psoriasis • Secondary to infectious diseases such as Lyme's disease, TB, toxoplasmosis, syphilis and herpes simplex, and herpes zoster viruses • Most cases are idiopathic	• Assess thorough history • Inspect eye • Referral to physician for testing and thorough eye exam

KEY FINDINGS	DIAGNOSTIC EVIDENCE
• The patient will have unexplained eye pain • The patient will possibly have blurred vision • The patient will have redness in the eye near the iris and a funny or small shaped pupil	• No diagnostic evidence available

Eye

Orbital Hematoma

HISTORY	MECHANISM OF INJURY	EVALUATION ESSENTIALS
• Patient reports blow to the eye and/or its surroundings • Acute onset • Pain identified with opening the eye	• Direct blow to the eye and/or eye area	• Assess patient for more serious injury including fracture and concussion • Inspect eye and surroundings • Evaluate eye motion

KEY FINDINGS	DIAGNOSTIC EVIDENCE
• The patient may have ecchymosis as well as associated swelling • More serious contusion will have subconjunctival hemorrhage and/or faulty vision	• No diagnostic evidence available

Eye

Ruptured Globe

HISTORY	MECHANISM OF INJURY	EVALUATION ESSENTIALS
• Patient reports severe pain • Acute onset • Patient complains of decreased visual acuity and diplopia	• Blow to eye by an object smaller than the eye orbit	• Assess pupils • Inspect for orbital leaking • Immediate referral to ophthalmologist required for full exam including ocular pressures

KEY FINDINGS	DIAGNOSTIC EVIDENCE
• History of direct blow to eye from smaller object such as a golf ball or racquetball • Severe pain and vision issues such as diplopia and decreased acuity • Patient will have irregular pupils, increased ocular pressure, and orbital leakage • Can lead to blindness	• No diagnostic evidence available

Eye

Stye and Blepharitis

HISTORY	MECHANISM OF INJURY	EVALUATION ESSENTIALS
• Patient reports painful pustule on the eyelid • Pain identified either at rest or with opening and closing eye	• Stye is a swollen sebaceous gland • Blepharitis is an infection of the eyelash follicle from staphylococcal organism by rubbing or dust particles	• Inspect eyelid

KEY FINDINGS	DIAGNOSTIC EVIDENCE
• There will be a red pustule on the upper or lower eyelid • The eyelid will be swollen	• No diagnostic evidence available

Eye

Subconjunctival Hematoma

HISTORY	MECHANISM OF INJURY	EVALUATION ESSENTIALS
• Patient reports having a red spot on the eye without any history of trauma • Acute onset • No pain or vision issue	• From rubbing eye in your sleep, with crying, or due to computer work • Forceful sneezing, coughing, vomiting, or lifting	• Inspect eye for redness • Inquire about other health history such as high blood pressure, uncontrolled diabetes, and hyperthyroidism

KEY FINDINGS	DIAGNOSTIC EVIDENCE
• A red spot will be seen on the conjunctiva that should last approximately 1 week • If taking an anticoagulant the subconjunctival hematoma would warrant a call to the primary care physician	• No diagnostic evidence available

Ear

Auricular Hematoma (Cauliflower Ear)

HISTORY	MECHANISM OF INJURY	EVALUATION ESSENTIALS
• Patient reports participating in wrestling, boxing, or rugby without headgear • Pain identified with trying to sleep on the affected side	• Compression of tissue in the ear to another surface • Shearing either single or repeated to the auricle	• Assess patient history • Inspect ear for hemorrhage and fluid accumulation • Refer to MD for aspiration if needed

KEY FINDINGS	DIAGNOSTIC EVIDENCE
• The patient will have obvious hematoma in the ear and will turn to keloid that is rounded, nodular, and firm if not attended to • The history will be consistent with participation in sport without protective headgear	• No diagnostic evidence available

Ear

Otitis Externa (Swimmer's Ear)

HISTORY	MECHANISM OF INJURY	EVALUATION ESSENTIALS
• Patient reports swimming in the history • Patient complains of pain, itching, discharge, and possible partial hearing loss	• Infection caused by *Pseudomonas aeruginosa*, a gram-negative bacillus • Water becomes trapped in the canal due to obstruction from cyst, bone growth, plugs of earwax, or swelling from allergens	• Assess external and internal ear with otoscope • Perform a test to differentiate otitis externa from otitis media by putting pressure over the tragus portion of the ear to put pressure on the canal, and if this causes pain, it is likely otitis externa versus otitis media

KEY FINDINGS	DIAGNOSTIC EVIDENCE
• The ear canal will be red and swollen and the tympanic membrane will be normal in color • Itching, discharge, and possible partial hearing loss may accompany the pain in the ear	• Otitis externa is usually diagnosed by physical examination, but the use of an ear swab may be used to confirm the source of the infection[14]

Ear

Otitis Media

HISTORY	MECHANISM OF INJURY	EVALUATION ESSENTIALS
• Patient reports intense pain in the ear, fluid draining from the ear canal, and transient hearing loss • Patient will complain of a systemic infection as well including fever, headache, anorexia, and nausea	• Accumulation of fluid in the middle ear caused by local and systemic infection and inflammation	• Assess patient history and symptoms • Inspect inner and outer ear with otoscope

KEY FINDINGS	DIAGNOSTIC EVIDENCE
• The tympanic membrane will be bulging and potentially bleeding • The patient will have pain, drainage, and a systemic infection	• Tympanic membrane bulging has a sensitivity of 51% and specificity of 97% for otitis media[15]

Ear

Tympanic Membrane Rupture

HISTORY	MECHANISM OF INJURY	EVALUATION ESSENTIALS
• Patient reports a loud pop followed by pain, nausea, dizziness, and potential vomiting • Patient complains of hearing loss • Acute onset • Pain identified with the pop	• Seen in contact and collision sports as well as with diving and water polo • A fall or slap to the unprotected ear • Sudden underwater variation • If a person has an ear infection and flies on an airplane, the abrupt change in cabin pressure can cause rupture as well	• Assess the external and internal ear with an otoscope • Continue follow up to prevent infection

KEY FINDINGS	DIAGNOSTIC EVIDENCE
• The history and physical exam will be consistent for acute onset and pop with pain • The patient will experience hearing loss, nausea, dizziness, and vomiting	• No diagnostic evidence available

Nose

Deviated Septum

HISTORY	MECHANISM OF INJURY	EVALUATION ESSENTIALS
• Patient reports nasal pain, potential bleeding, and history of some trauma to the nose • Acute onset	• Trauma to the nose • Compression or lateral trauma	• Assess the patient fully for fracture or other injury • Inspect the external and internal nose if possible • Refer to MD for treatment

KEY FINDINGS	DIAGNOSTIC EVIDENCE
• There is obvious deformity at the nose • The patient will have pain and possibly bleeding with the history of trauma	• The use of an endoscope can help confirm diagnosis of a deviated septum[16]

Nose

Epistaxis

HISTORY	MECHANISM OF INJURY	EVALUATION ESSENTIALS
• Patient reports having a bloody nose	• Direct blow to the nose with varying degrees of contusion to the septum • Categorized as anterior originating from the nasal septum or posterior originating from the lateral wall • Anterior more common resulting from direct blow, sinus infection, high humidity, allergy, foreign body lodged in the nose, or other serious facial or head injury	• Assess inside of the nose if possible with penlight and speculum • Inspect for more serious injury

KEY FINDINGS	DIAGNOSTIC EVIDENCE
• The patient will be bleeding from the nose • There will not be a deformity at the nose	• No diagnostic evidence available

Mouth and Jaw

Mandibular Luxation

HISTORY	MECHANISM OF INJURY	EVALUATION ESSENTIALS
• Patient reports locked open jaw • Acute onset • Pain identified with side blow to the jaw	• Side blow to an open mouth	• Assess AROM and PROM • Inspect inside of mouth and jaw • Refer to rule out fracture

KEY FINDINGS	DIAGNOSTIC EVIDENCE
• The patient will not be able to move jaw; it is locked open • The patient will have pain and malocclusion of the teeth	• Radiographs and CT may be required to determine the presence of a fracture and the need for surgical management[17]

Mouth and Jaw

Temporomandibular Joint Dysfunction

HISTORY	MECHANISM OF INJURY	EVALUATION ESSENTIALS
• Patient reports headache, vertigo, inflammation, and neck pain • Chronic onset • Pain identified with opening and closing mouth, talking, and chewing	• A disk-condyle derangement • Can progress to deterioration of the posterior stabilizing structures and anterior dislocation of the disk	• Assess active and passive motion at the jaw • Inspect the inside of the mouth as well • Assess joint mobility • Evaluate muscle strength

KEY FINDINGS	DIAGNOSTIC EVIDENCE
• The patient will have audible click with both opening and closing mouth • Tenderness to palpation at the TMJ • The patient will likely be muscle guarding and have palpable trigger points • The joint will either be hyper- or hypomobile with decreased ROM	• MRI is 95% accurate in determining disc position and form. It is the most common choice of imaging for TMJ dysfunction.[18] • Ultrasonography (sensitivity 76%, specificity 82%)[19]

Mouth and Jaw

Tooth Luxations

HISTORY	MECHANISM OF INJURY	EVALUATION ESSENTIALS
• Patient reports a loose or totally dislodged tooth • Acute onset • Patient will have little to no pain but feels like the tooth is different	• Impact either direct or indirect to the jaw or tooth	• Assess patient for concussion • Inspect mouth and all teeth

KEY FINDINGS	DIAGNOSTIC EVIDENCE
• The patient will still have the tooth or teeth in place; however it will be either forward or backward in relation to the other teeth • The history will be in line with the severity of the injury to the tooth	• No diagnostic evidence available

Mouth and Jaw

Trigeminal Neuralgia

HISTORY	MECHANISM OF INJURY	EVALUATION ESSENTIALS
• Patient reports episodes of extreme sporadic, sudden burning or shock-like face pain lasting from a few seconds to 2 minutes per episode	• Compression of the nerve by a blood vessel as it exits the base of the brain • It may be part of the normal aging process • Can occur in people with MS, tumor or can be idiopathic in nature	• Assess patient history • Refer to a neurologist

KEY FINDINGS	DIAGNOSTIC EVIDENCE
• The patient has excruciating pain episodes • Patient may have family history of same painful episodes • Patient may have MS or a tumor • Patient may experience numbness or tingling • Patient may experience an increase in frequency with time; this rarely occurs at night during sleep	• MRI may be used to determine the source of symptoms[20]

Paper Patient: Revisited

You should have been able to rule out several conditions secondary to knowing what the various head injuries are. Your differentials should have been mTBI, subdural, and epidural hematoma.

Learning Activities: Practice Case

Use the blank templates provided in the appendices to write out a differential diagnosis map and clinical findings overview for the case provided below. When working with paper patients it is tempting to try to jump to "the answer" and come to a diagnosis. However, the visual learning approach to differential diagnosis is designed to help you consider all the possibilities for the information provided. Good luck.

Paper Patient: Facial Injury in a Baseball Player

History

Jake is a 20-year-old baseball player who slid into third base head first and was hit by a ball that went straight down the line. He was found to be conscious when you got to the base. He reports pain in the nose and cheek on the right side, and he is bleeding from the right nostril. He denies neck pain.

Physical Exam

Your physical exam on the field reveals no tenderness over the cervical spine. He does not have retro- or anterograde amnesia. The patient denies a headache or other symptoms of concussion. He has tenderness to palpation over the mid portion of the nose and the cheekbone off to the right side. The eyes are WNL. Cervical ROM was WNL. The patient is bleeding from the right nostril and it slows down after you get the patient to the dugout. The patient rates his pain as 7/10.

References

1. Behavioral Risk Factor Surveillance System: Exercise. Centers for Disease Control and Prevention; 2006. Available at: http://apps.nccd.cdc.gov/brfss/. Accessed June 12, 2014.
2. Daneshvar DH, et al. The epidemiology of sport-related concussion. *Clinics in sports medicine 30.1* (2011): 1.

3. Langlois JA, Rutland-Brown W, Wald MM. The epidemiologyand impact of traumatic brain injury: a brief overview. *J Head Trauma Rehabil* 2006;21:375–378.
4. Gessell LM, Fields SK, Collins CL, Dick RW, Comstock RD. Concussions among United States high school and collegiate athletes. *J Athl Train* 2007;42:495–503.
5. Lincoln AE, Caswell SV, Almquist JL, Dunn RE, Norris JB, Hinton RY. Trends in concussion incidence in high school sports: a prospective 11-year study. *Am J Sports Med.* 2011;39:958-963.
6. Faul M, Xu L, Wald MM, Coronado VG. *Traumatic Brain Injury in the United States: Emergency Department Visits, Hospitalizations and Deaths 2002-2006.* US Department of Health and Human Services; Mar, 2010.
7. Finkelstein E, Corso P, Miller T. *The Incidence and Economic Burden of Injuries in the United States.* New York, NY: Oxford University Press; 2006.
8. McCrory P, Meeuwisse WH, Aubry M, et al. Consensus statement on concussion in sport: the 4th International Conference on Concussion in Sport held in Zurich, November 2012. *British Journal of Sports Medicine.* 2013;47.5:250-258.
9. Guskiewicz KM, Bruce SL, Cantu RC, et al. Recommendations on management of sport-related concussion: summary of the National Athletic Trainers' Association position statement. *Neurosurgery.* 2004;55(4):891-896.
10. McCrory P, Johnston K, Meeuwisse W, et al. Summary and agreement statement of the 2nd International Conference on Concussion in Sport, Prague 2004. *British Journal of Sports Medicine.* 2005:39.4;196-204.
11. Kubal WS. Updated imaging of traumatic brain injury. *Radiol Clin North Am.* 2012;50(1):15-41.
12. Pointinger H, Sarahrudi K, Poeschl G, Munk P. Electroencephalography in primary diagnosis of mild head trauma. *Brain Inj.* 2002;16(9):799-805.
13. Wipperman JL, Dorsch JN. Evaluation and management of corneal abrasions. *Am Fam Physician.* 2013;87(2):114-120.
14. Kaushik V, Malik T, Saeed SR. Interventions for acute otitis externa. *Cochrane Database Syst Rev.* 2010;(1).
15. Lieberthal AS, Carroll AE, Chonmaitree T, et al. The diagnosis and management of acute otitis media. *Pediatrics.* 2013;131(3).
16. Higuera S, Lee EI, Cole P, Hollier LH Jr, Stal S. Nasal trauma and the deviated nose. *Plast Reconstr Surg.* 2007;120(7 Suppl 2):64S-75S.
17. Akinbami BO. Evaluation of the mechanism and principles of management of temporomandibular joint dislocation. Systematic review of literature and a proposed new classification of temporomandibular joint dislocation. *Head Face Med.* 2011;7:10.
18. Maizlin ZV, Nutiu N, Dent PB, et al. Displacement of the temporomandibular joint disk: correlation between clinical findings and MRI characteristics. *J Can Dent Assoc.* 2010;76:a3.
19. Li C, Su N, Yang X, Yang X, Shi Z, Li L. Ultrasonography for detection of disc displacement of temporomandibular joint: a systematic review and meta-analysis. *J Oral Maxillofac Surg.* 2012;70(6):1300-1309.
20. van Kleef M, van Genderen WE, Narouze S, et 1. Trigeminal neuralgia. *Pain Pract.* 2009;9(4):252-259.

11

The Abdomen and Thorax

Injuries to organ systems and the cardiorespiratory structures of the abdomen and thorax represent a small percentage of the sports injuries seen by clinicians. Despite these injuries being relatively uncommon, the consequences may be catastrophic if they are not properly recognized or if their recognition is delayed. In contrast to athletic injuries of other organ systems, thoracoabdominal injuries generally result from either rapid deceleration or high-energy impact to the thorax or abdomen.[1] Athletes involved in high-speed sports (eg, bicycling, skiing, motorized events), high-altitude sports (eg, bungee jumping, parachuting, rock climbing) or high-energy contact sports (eg, football, hockey, boxing) are at particular risk. While these high-speed sports carry greater risk, thoracoabdominal injuries can occur in any athlete in any sport.

There are several examples of the seriousness of injuries to the abdomen and thorax. A review of kidney injuries in the National Football League over 8 seasons[2] identified an average of 2.7 cases per season, with the injury rate for games 10 times greater than practice. Kidney contusions were the most common injury (n=42), followed by kidney laceration (n=6). A report of skiing injuries over a 12-year period at one North American ski resort medical center found a total of 18 splenic ruptures: 6 of these injuries were high-speed collisions with trees, lift towers, or other solid objects; 12 were low-speed falls to skiers who skied down the mountain without assistance and later developed symptoms requiring treatment at a hospital.[3] Meehan and Mannix[4] reported on a 10-year study of emergency room visits examining

Winterstein AP, Clark SV. *The Athletic Trainer's Guide to Differential Diagnosis (pp 357-388).*

life-threatening injuries and found that 14% of all life-threatening injuries were sport related. A higher percentage of these injuries were in children (32%) compared with adults (9%). Samples of diagnoses in the survey that qualify as life-threatening include traumatic pneumothorax and hemothorax, liver lacerations, spleen lacerations, aortic rupture, gastric/duodenal rupture, and commotio cordis/heart contusion. Although injuries to the head and neck represent a much higher level of catastrophic outcome, injuries to the abdomen and thorax cannot be taken for granted.

Clinicians responsible for evaluating possible injuries to the abdomen and thorax have a heightened responsibility to evaluate and manage these injuries with great care so that a potentially catastrophic problem is not overlooked. The differential diagnosis map works well with the division of the abdomen and thorax into 4 logical quadrants. Clinicians can use the differential diagnosis map, coupled with their knowledge of the underlying anatomy, pain referral patterns, and injury signs and symptoms, to guide them as they determine a diagnosis and course of action.

Paper Patient: Thorax/Abdominal Injury in a Football Player

History

Rob is a 15-year-old football player. During a game, he landed on the football, and the opposing team's player landed on top of him on his right side. You perform an exam on the field.

Physical Exam

The patient has tenderness to palpation over ribs 8 to 12 that does not extend much beyond the midline of the ribcage. He complains of more pain with inhalation than exhalation and no trouble breathing. There is no palpable or observable deformity. He denies nausea, chills, or lightheadedness. He is not coughing up blood or other fluid. The patient rates his pain as 8/10 on the visual analog scale of 0 to 10.

Clinical Decisions

Using the information from your clinical exam, ask yourself these questions to guide your clinical decision making:

- What is your differential diagnosis?
- What key findings do you see to help guide your differential?

- What are the possible injuries associated with ribcage pain?

Start with a review of the anatomy maps and a thorough consideration of the possible injuries and conditions that are common to the abdomen and thorax. Use the differential diagnosis maps to guide your thought process and organize the possibilities. The organized synthesis of this information is the essence of clinical decision making.

Anatomy Map: Viscera

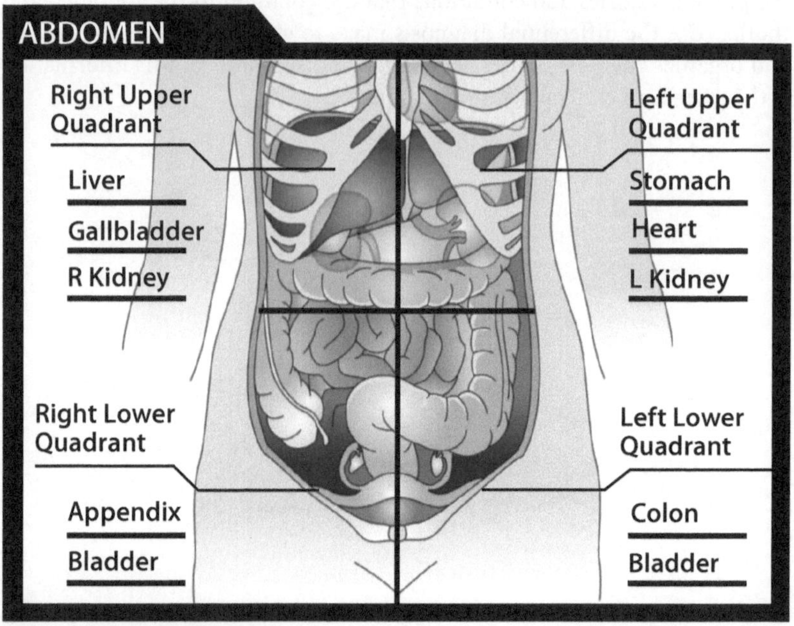

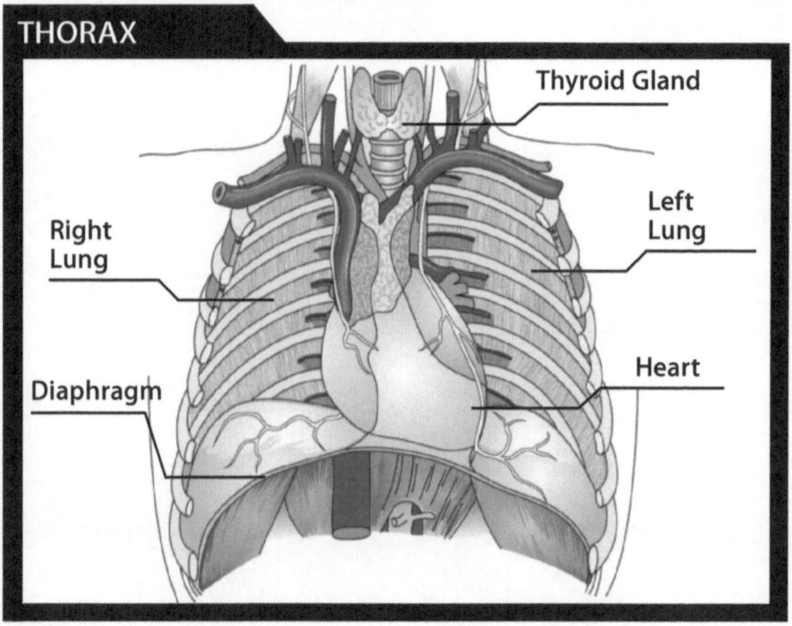

Anatomy Map: Thorax

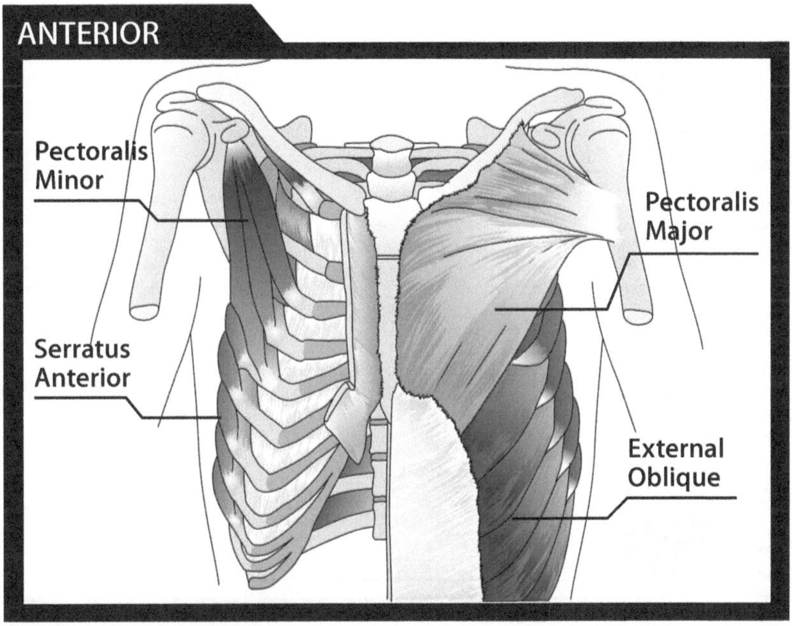

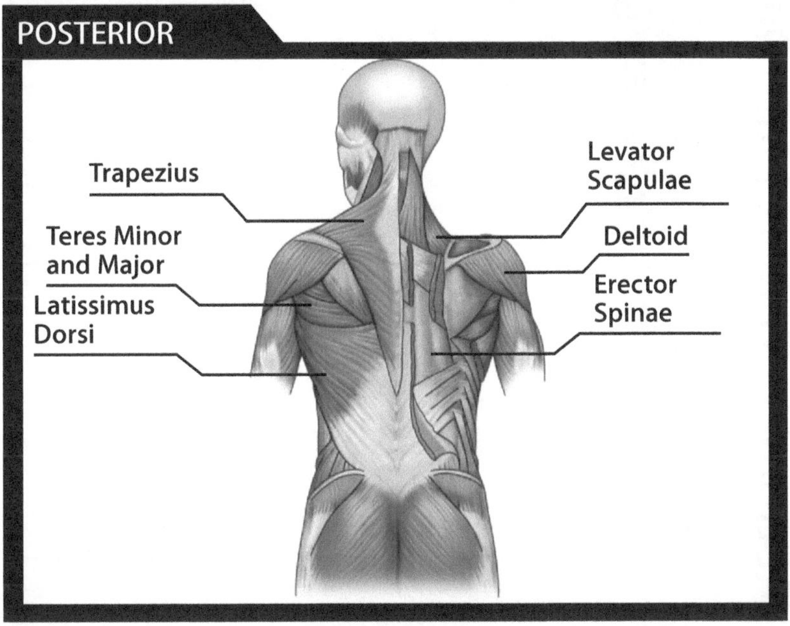

Abdomen/Thorax Map: Differential Diagnosis by Quadrant

UPPER RIGHT

- Costochondral Injury
- Hemothorax
- Kidney Contusion
- Kidney Stones
- Pneumothorax
- Solar Plexus Injury

UPPER LEFT

- Commotio Cordis
- Costochondral Injury
- Hemothorax
- Kidney Stones
- Pneumothorax
- Solar Plexus Injury
- Splenic Enlargement/ Rupture

LOWER RIGHT

- Abdominal Strain
- Appendicitis
- Hernia
- Psoas Strain

LOWER LEFT

- Abdominal Strain
- Hernia
- Psoas Strain

Injuries to the Thorax

Rib and Sternum Fractures

COMMON FRACTURES

- **Rib Fractures**
    - The most common thoracic injury; thought to be present in 10% of all traumatic injuries.
    - Fractures typically affect the fifth through ninth ribs. This may be due to the fact that the shoulder girdle protects the upper ribs and the lower ribs are relatively mobile.
    - While rib fractures can produce significant morbidity, the diagnosis of associated complications (eg, pneumothorax, hemothorax, cardiovascular injury) may have a more significant clinical impact.
    - Radiographs are specific but not very sensitive for undisplaced fractures, and clinical examination is sensitive but not specific.
- **Multiple Rib Fractures**
    - The presence of multiple rib fractures (3 or more) is associated with increased risk of respiratory complications.
- **Stress Fractures to the Rib**
    - Ribs are overall an uncommon site for stress fracture in the general population.
    - Some sport activities, notably rowing, place significant overuse stress on the ribs and stress fractures are not uncommon in this circumstance.
- **Sternum Fractures**
    - Occurs in 5% to 8% of people who experience significant blunt chest trauma; common in vehicle accidents.
    - Can occur in sport with direct blows; injuries to underlying organs are primary concern.

Adapted from Bansidhar BJ, Lagares-Garcia JA, Miller SL. Clinical rib fractures: are follow-up chest X-rays a waste of resources? *Am Surg* 2002; 68(5):449-453.

Abdominal Pain

Acute Abdomen/Warnings/Physical Exam

CONSIDERATIONS

- **Acute Abdomen** refers to a sudden, severe pain in the abdomen that is less than 24 hours in duration, which suggests a disease or injury that possibly threatens life and demands an immediate or urgent diagnosis for early treatment.
- **Warning signs** when evaluating abdominal pain are as follows.
    - Vomiting blood or black material (like coffee grounds)
    - Fever of 101 degrees Fahrenheit (38.3 degrees Celsius) or higher with associated abdominal pain
    - Persistent vomiting (unable to keep fluids down for more than 24 to 36 hours; less in younger athletes)
- **Referred pain patterns** (examples)
    - Left shoulder pain: possible spleen injury
    - Right scapular/shoulder pain: possible liver injury
    - Left jaw and arm pain: possible cardiac event
- **Abdominal Exam** (palpation)
    - Rigidity: muscle guarding may indicate peritoneal irritation
    - Rebound tenderness: abdominal pain upon release of palpation; common with appendicitis
- **Location of Pain and Common Imaging Techniques**
    - Right upper quadrant—Ultrasonography
    - Left upper quadrant—CT
    - Right lower quadrant—CT + IV contrast
    - Left lower quadrant—CT + oral and IV media
    - Suprapubic—Ultrasonography

Abdominal Pain

General Abdominal Evaluation

EVALUATION SCHEME

- **History**
  - Pain, onset, duration, quality, severity, and radiation
  - Associated symptoms: nausea, vomiting, diarrhea, constipation, fever, fatigue, and painful urination
  - Aggravating and alleviating factors
  - Appetite and food tolerance
  - Bowel habits
- **Observation**
  - Visible ecchymosis
  - Tone
  - Color
- **Auscultation** (do prior to percussion and palpation)
  - Bowel sounds
  - Vascular sounds
- **Percussion**
  - Percuss the 4 quadrants
- **Palpation**
  - Light palpation to assess tenderness in the quadrants
  - Deeper palpation for pain and masses
  - Direct palpation of spleen, liver, kidneys, and McBurney's point

Adapted from Cuppett M, Walsh KM. *General Medical Conditions in the Athlete*. 2nd ed. St. Louis, MO: Elsevier Mosby Inc; 2012.

Abdominal Pain

Common Diagnostic Possibilities by Location

LOCATION / CONDITIONS

- **Epigastric**—Peptic ulcer disease, gastric reflux
- **Right Upper Quadrant**—Liver, gall bladder, urinary tract infection
- **Left Upper Quadrant**—Spleen, Gastric ulcer
- **Right Lower Quadrant**—Appendicitis
- **Left Lower Quadrant**—Constipation, Meckel's diverticulum
- **Suprapubic**—Urinary tract infection, sexually transmitted infections

Note: The epigastric region is located in the central portion ofabdomen just inferior to the sternum and above the umbilicus. The suprapubic region is located between the umbilicus and the pubic symphysis.

Clinical Assessment of Abdomen and Thorax

Upper Right Quadrant Pain

Costochondral Injury

HISTORY	MECHANISM OF INJURY	EVALUATION ESSENTIALS
• Patient reports pain in the chest or with twisting • Acute onset • Pain identified with breathing, coughing, laughing, or sneezing	• Violent injury to the chest or rib cage forcing a stretch at the Costochondral junction • Piling on or crushing injury such as in rugby or football	• Assess point tenderness and have patient cough or laugh • Inspect chest area for swelling • Evaluate AROM and PROM • Evaluate muscle strength

KEY FINDINGS	DIAGNOSTIC EVIDENCE
• Specific tenderness over the costochondral joint • Logical history associated with clinical findings • Initial injury may present with palpable defect	• No diagnostic evidence available

Upper Right Quadrant Pain

Hemothorax

HISTORY

- Patient reports a blow to the chest, pain, and difficulty breathing
- Acute onset

MECHANISM OF INJURY

- A violent blow to or compression of the chest causing the lung to hemorrhage

EVALUATION ESSENTIALS

- Assess vitals including pulse, respiratory rate, and breathing
- Inspect chest for uniformity when breathing for sign of rib fracture that may accompany the hemothorax

KEY FINDINGS

- The patient will have labored breathing and pain and look cyanotic
- The patient will cough up frothy blood and possibly present with signs of shock
- The history and physical exam will be consistent

DIAGNOSTIC EVIDENCE

- Radiographs and CT are often used to determine extent of injury[5]

Upper Right Quadrant Pain

Kidney Contusion

HISTORY	MECHANISM OF INJURY	EVALUATION ESSENTIALS
• Patient reports hematuria along with nausea and vomiting • Acute onset • Pain will be posterior possibly radiating forward	• A direct blow to the back or abdomen	• Assess point tenderness • Inspect urine for hematuria by having patient urinate 2 to 3 times • Evaluate AROM and PROM

KEY FINDINGS	DIAGNOSTIC EVIDENCE
• The patient will have severe pain posterior possibly radiating forward around the trunk into the lower abdominal region. They may present with signs of shock. Like other organs, kidneys refer pain to the outside of the body. • The patient will likely complain of nausea and vomiting • If there is blood in the urine, a referral is necessary	• CT is the gold standard for assessing the kidneys[6]

Upper Right Quadrant Pain

Kidney Stones

HISTORY	MECHANISM OF INJURY	EVALUATION ESSENTIALS
• Patient reports nausea and vomiting and difficulty getting comfortable • Acute onset • Pain is sudden, sharp, and severe	• Small crystals that form in the kidney, and etiology is not precisely known • Most common type is calcium when too much calcium combines with other waste products in the urine	• Assess point tenderness and pain pattern as well as frequency of urination • Inspect urine for hematuria

KEY FINDINGS	DIAGNOSTIC EVIDENCE
• The patient will have severe pain in the low back or in the flank on one side and shoots towards the groin on that same side • The patient will likely complain of nausea and vomiting and present with skin that is cool, clammy, pale, and sweaty • Urination will be frequent with burning and possibly with blood	• Ultrasound (sensitivity 45%, specificity 88%)[7] • CT (sensitivity ~100%, specificity ~100%)[8]

Upper Right Quadrant Pain

Pneumothorax

HISTORY	MECHANISM OF INJURY	EVALUATION ESSENTIALS
• Patient reports a blow to the chest • Acute onset • There is pain, difficulty breathing, and anoxia	• A blow to the chest causing the pleural cavity to become filled with air that has entered through an opening in the chest. The negatively pressured pleural cavity fills with air, and the lung on that side collapses. • A secondary complication of surgery particularly for the first rib	• Assess vitals including pulse, respiratory rate, and breathing • Inspect chest for uniformity or breath sounds

KEY FINDINGS	DIAGNOSTIC EVIDENCE
• The patient will have labored breathing and potentially pain and anoxia. • The history and physical exam will be consistent	• Radiographs and CT are often used to determine extent of injury[5]

Upper Right Quadrant Pain

Solar Plexus Injury

HISTORY	MECHANISM OF INJURY	EVALUATION ESSENTIALS
• Patient reports a blow to the chest/abdomen • Patient states that they got the wind knocked out of them once they are calmed down • Acute onset	• A violent blow to or compression of the solar plexus (sympathetic celiac plexus) that produces a paralysis of the diaphragm	• Assess breathing and then other vitals • Inspect chest for uniformity when breathing for sign of rib fracture

KEY FINDINGS	DIAGNOSTIC EVIDENCE
• The patient will be unable to inhale, and demonstrate a bit of hysteria due to fear of not being able to breathe and hyperventilate. • The history and physical exam will be consistent	• No diagnostic evidence available

Upper Left Quadrant Pain

Commotio Cordis

HISTORY	MECHANISM OF INJURY	EVALUATION ESSENTIALS
• Acute onset • History of direct blow to the chest	• Traumatic blunt impact to the chest resulting in cardiac arrest • In about half the cases, death is immediate, while in others there is a brief period of consciousness before collapse	• Assess ABCs • Inspect chest • ECG will reveal ventricular fibrillation

KEY FINDINGS	DIAGNOSTIC EVIDENCE
• History is consistent with blunt trauma to the chest • The patient will be in ventricular fibrillation if they are conscious, otherwise they will have already died	• 78% of cases occur in athletes under 18 years old • 95% of cases are male[9]

Upper Left Quadrant Pain

Costochondral Injury

HISTORY	MECHANISM OF INJURY	EVALUATION ESSENTIALS
• Patient reports pain in the chest or with twisting • Acute onset • Pain identified with breathing, coughing, laughing, or sneezing	• Violent injury to the chest or rib cage forcing a stretch at the Costochondral junction • Piling on or crushing injury such as in rugby or football	• Assess point tenderness and have patient cough or laugh • Inspect chest area for swelling • Evaluate AROM and PROM • Evaluate muscle strength

KEY FINDINGS	DIAGNOSTIC EVIDENCE
• The patient will have pain with coughing, sneezing, or laughing • There may or may not be swelling • The patient will have pain anytime the muscles are stretched across the chest • Breathing will be painful but not difficult	• No diagnostic evidence available

Upper Left Quadrant Pain

Hemothorax

HISTORY	MECHANISM OF INJURY	EVALUATION ESSENTIALS
• Patient reports a blow to the chest, pain, and difficulty breathing • Acute onset	• A violent blow to or compression of the chest causing the lung to hemorrhage	• Assess vitals including pulse, respiratory rate, and breathing • Inspect chest for uniformity when breathing for sign of rib fracture that may accompany the hemothorax

KEY FINDINGS	DIAGNOSTIC EVIDENCE
• The patient will have labored breathing and pain and look cyanotic. • The patient will cough up frothy blood and possibly present with signs of shock • The history and physical exam will be consistent	• Radiographs and CT are often used to determine extent of injury[5]

Upper Left Quadrant Pain

Kidney Stones

HISTORY	MECHANISM OF INJURY	EVALUATION ESSENTIALS
• Patient reports nausea and vomiting and difficulty getting comfortable • Acute onset • Pain is sudden, sharp, and severe	• Small crystals that form in the kidney and etiology is not precisely known • Most common type is calcium when too much calcium combines with other waste products in the urine.	• Assess point tenderness and pain pattern as well as frequency of urination • Inspect urine for hematuria

KEY FINDINGS	DIAGNOSTIC EVIDENCE
• The patient will have severe pain in the low back or in the flank on one side and shoots towards the groin on that same side • The patient will likely complain of nausea and vomiting and present with skin that is cool, clammy, pale, and sweaty • Urination will be frequent with burning and possibly with blood	• Ultrasound (sensitivity 45%, specificity 88%)[7] • CT (sensitivity ~100%, specificity ~100%)[8]

Upper Left Quadrant Pain

Pneumothorax

HISTORY	MECHANISM OF INJURY	EVALUATION ESSENTIALS
• Patient reports a blow to the chest • Acute onset • There is pain, difficulty breathing, and anoxia	• A blow to the chest causing the pleural cavity to become filled with air that has entered through an opening in the chest. The negatively pressured pleural cavity fills with air, the lung on that side collapses. • A secondary complication of surgery particularly for the first rib	• Assess vitals including pulse, respiratory rate, and breathing • Inspect chest for uniformity or breath sounds

KEY FINDINGS	DIAGNOSTIC EVIDENCE
• The patient will have labored breathing and potentially pain and anoxia. • The history and physical exam will be consistent	• Radiographs and CT are often used to determine extent of injury[5]

Upper Left Quadrant Pain

Solar Plexus Injury

HISTORY	MECHANISM OF INJURY	EVALUATION ESSENTIALS
• Patient reports a blow to the chest/abdomen • Patient states that he or she got the wind knocked out of him or her once he or she is calmed down • Acute onset	• A violent blow to or compression of the solar plexus (sympathetic celiac plexus) that produces a paralysis of the diaphragm	• Assess breathing and then other vitals • Inspect chest for uniformity in breathing patterns • Inspect and palpate for signs of rib fracture

KEY FINDINGS	DIAGNOSTIC EVIDENCE
• The patient will be unable to inhale and demonstrate a bit of hysteria due to fear of not being able to breathe and hyperventilate • The history and physical exam will be consistent	• No diagnostic evidence available

Upper Left Quadrant Pain

Splenic Enlargement/Rupture

HISTORY	MECHANISM OF INJURY	EVALUATION ESSENTIALS
• Patient reports being in a car accident or a direct blow to the left upper quadrant • Acute onset • Pain identified in the abdomen	• Car accident • Direct blow to the upper left quadrant	• Assess patient for shock • Palpate abdomen • Perform abdominal percussion • Assess for Kehr's sign

KEY FINDINGS	DIAGNOSTIC EVIDENCE
• The patient may be in shock • The abdomen will be rigid • The patient may have nausea and report vomiting • The history and physical exam will be consistent with abdominal trauma and pain	• CT is the most common form of imaging used for diagnosis[10]

Lower Right Quadrant Pain

Abdominal Strain

HISTORY	MECHANISM OF INJURY	EVALUATION ESSENTIALS
• Patient reports abdominal pain • Acute onset • Pain identified with the motion of the abdominal muscle injured	• Overstretch of the muscle with twisting motion • Maximal contraction in a shorted position and then stretched	• Assess tenderness to palpation • Inspect abdomen for ecchymosis • Assess AROM and PROM • Evaluate muscle strength

KEY FINDINGS	DIAGNOSTIC EVIDENCE
• The patient will have immediate abdominal pain in the strained muscle • It will be hard to flex the muscle due to pain • There will likely be spasm of the injured muscle • May find swelling and ecchymosis	• Ultrasonography and MRI can be used to confirm diagnosis[11]

Lower Right Quadrant Pain

Appendicitis

HISTORY	MECHANISM OF INJURY	EVALUATION ESSENTIALS
• Patient reports nausea, vomiting, and fever • Acute or chronic onset • Pain identified in the lower right abdomen	• A fecal obstruction • Lymph swelling • Carcinoid tumor • Peritonitis or bacterial infections are complications of rupture	• Assess vitals including oral temperature • Inspect abdomen for pain at McBurney's point • Evaluate abdomen with percussion also to assess rigidity

KEY FINDINGS	DIAGNOSTIC EVIDENCE
• The symptoms range in severity and can progress from mild to severe pain, and later, cramps may localize pain in the right side • The abdomen will be rigid with tenderness over McBurney's point • This can be life threatening	• CT (sensitivity 94%, specificity 94%) • Ultrasound (sensitivity 83%, specificity 93%)[12] • MRI (sensitivity 97%, specificity 95%)[13]

Lower Right Quadrant Pain

Hernia

HISTORY

- Patient reports a feeling of weakness or pulling sensation in the groin
- Chronic onset
- Pain identified with coughing, sneezing, or laughing

MECHANISM OF INJURY

- Is acquired; developed after birth or congenital; developed before birth
- Femoral is more common for females and inguinal for males

EVALUATION ESSENTIALS

- Assess abdomen for protrusion near inguinal canal or in the femoral triangle
- Inspect abdomen for swelling in standing

KEY FINDINGS

- The patient may have a strain or blow to the groin area that produced pain and prolonged discomfort.
- The patient will have a protrusion that is increased with coughing or bearing down.

DIAGNOSTIC EVIDENCE

- Ultrasound (sensitivity 86%, specificity 77%)
- CT (sensitivity 80%, specificity 65%)[14]
- MRI (sensitivity 94.5%)[15]

Lower Right Quadrant Pain

Psoas Strain

HISTORY	MECHANISM OF INJURY	EVALUATION ESSENTIALS
• Patient reports tightness in the anterior hip • Acute onset • Pain identified with flexing the hip	• Increasing mileage too quickly or excessive speed workout • Excessive eccentric load to the psoas	• Assess hip flexor tightness with Thomas test • Inspect anterior hip for swelling or ecchymosis • Evaluate muscle strength

KEY FINDINGS	DIAGNOSTIC EVIDENCE
• The patient will not have feelings of malaise or low-grade fever • The patient will have pain in the anterior hip and a history consistent with muscle strain	• No diagnostic evidence available

Lower Left Quadrant Pain

Abdominal Strain

HISTORY	MECHANISM OF INJURY	EVALUATION ESSENTIALS
• Patient reports abdominal pain • Acute onset • Pain identified with the motion of the abdominal muscle injured	• Overstretch of the muscle with twisting motion • Maximal contraction in a shorted position and then stretched	• Assess tenderness to palpation • Inspect abdomen for ecchymosis • Assess AROM and PROM • Evaluate muscle strength

KEY FINDINGS	DIAGNOSTIC EVIDENCE
• The patient will have immediate abdominal pain in the strained muscle • It will be hard to flex the muscle due to pain • There will likely be spasm of the injured muscle • May find swelling and ecchymosis	• Ultrasonography and MRI can be used to confirm diagnosis[11]

Lower Left Quadrant Pain

Hernia

HISTORY	MECHANISM OF INJURY	EVALUATION ESSENTIALS
• Patient reports a feeling of weakness or pulling sensation in the groin • Chronic onset • Pain identified with coughing, sneezing, or laughing	• Is acquired; developed after birth or congenital; developed before birth • Femoral is more common for females and inguinal for males	• Assess abdomen for protrusion near inguinal canal or in the femoral triangle • Inspect abdomen for swelling in standing

KEY FINDINGS	DIAGNOSTIC EVIDENCE
• The patient may have a strain or blow to the groin area that produced pain and prolonged discomfort • The patient will have a protrusion that is increased with coughing or bearing down	• Ultrasound (sensitivity 86%, specificity 77%) • CT (sensitivity 80%, specificity 65%)[14] • MRI (sensitivity 94.5%)[15]

Lower Left Quadrant Pain

Psoas Strain

HISTORY	MECHANISM OF INJURY	EVALUATION ESSENTIALS
• Patient reports tightness in the anterior hip • Acute onset • Pain identified with flexing the hip	• Increasing mileage too quickly or excessive speed workout • Excessive eccentric load to the psoas	• Assess hip flexor tightness with Thomas test • Inspect anterior hip for swelling or ecchymosis • Evaluate muscle strength

KEY FINDINGS	DIAGNOSTIC EVIDENCE
• The patient will not have feelings of malaise or low-grade fever • The patient will have pain in the anterior hip and a history consistent with muscle strain	• No diagnostic evidence available

Paper Patient: Revisited

You should have been able to rule out several conditions secondary to knowing what structures are at the right upper and lower quadrants. Your differential should have been rib contusion, rib fracture versus possible liver laceration.

Learning Activities: Practice Case

Use the blank templates provided in the Appendices to write out a differential diagnosis map and clinical findings overview for the case provided below. When working with paper patients, it is tempting to try to jump to "the answer" and come to a diagnosis. However, the visual learning approach to differential diagnosis is designed to help you consider all the possibilities for the information provided. Refer to Chapter 12 for additional learning activities.

Paper Patient: Abdominal Pain in a Recreational Softball Player

History

Julie is a 30-year-old recreational softball player who was injured when a runner collided with her while she was making a play at second base. She fell to the ground and states that she felt as if she "got the wind knocked out of her." Julie completed the next inning and reported pain in her abdomen while sitting in the dugout later in the game. She described some nausea and lightheadedness. She was removed from play and evaluated immediately. Julie states she is having pain in the left side of her rib cage and abdomen. She also describes pain in the left shoulder.

Physical Exam

The physical exam reveals that the patient appears pale and there is tenderness in the upper region of the abdomen, with some tenderness in the upper left quadrant. There is a palpable tension in the abdomen. There is also tenderness in the left rib cage region. Blood pressure is 100/75, which is lower than normal for this patient.

References

1. Amaral JF. Thoracoabdominal injuries in the athlete. *Clin Sports Med.* 1997;16(4):739-753.
2. Brophy RH. Kidney injuries in professional American football: Implications for management of an athlete with one functioning kidney. *Am J Sports Med.* 2008;36(1):85-90.
3. Sartorelli KH, Pilcher DB, Rogers FB. Patterns of splenic injuries seen in skiers. *Injury.* 1995;26(1):43-46.
4. Meehan WP, Mannix R. A substantial proportion of life-threatening injuries are sport-related. *Pediatr Emerg Care.* 2013;29(5): 624-627.
5. Feden JP. Closed lung trauma. *Clin Sports Med.* 2013;32(2):255-265.
6. Viola TA. Closed kidney injury. *Clin Sports Med.* 2013;32(2):219-227.
7. Ray AA, Ghiculete D, Pace KT, Honey RJ. Limitations to ultrasound in the detection and measurement of urinary tract calculi. *Urology.* 2010;76(2):295-300.
8. Vrtiska TJ, Krambeck AE, McCollough CH, et al. Imaging evaluation and treatment of nephrolithiasis: An update. *Minn Med.* 2010;93(8):48-51.
9. Bock JS, Benitez RM. Blunt cardiac injury. *Cardiol Clin.* 2012;30(4):545-555.
10. Raikhlin A, Baerlocher MO, Asch MR, Myers A. Imaging and transcatheter arterial embolization for traumatic splenic injuries: Review of the literature. *Can J Surg.* 2008;51(6):464-472.
11. Obaid H, Nealon A, Connell D. Sonographic appearance of side strain injury. *AJR Am J Roentgenol.* 2008;191(6):W264-267.
12. Rybkin AV, Thoeni RF. Current concepts in imaging of appendicitis. R*adiol Clin North Am.* 2007;45(3):411-422.
13. Barger RL Jr, Nandalur KR. Diagnostic performance of magnetic resonance imaging in the detection of appendicitis in adults: A meta-analysis. *Acad Radiol.* 2010;17(10):1211-1216.
14. Robinson A, Light D, Kasim A, Nice C. A systematic review and meta-analysis of the role of radiology in the diagnosis of occult inguinal hernia. *Surg Endosc.* 2013;27(1):11-18.
15. van den Berg JC. Inguinal hernias: MRI and ultrasound. *Semin Ultrasound CT MR.* 2002;23(2):156-173.

12

Learning Activities

Paper Patients and Case Studies

This chapter provides students with a random collection of Paper Patients. These short case studies are designed to provide learners with multiple opportunities to create their own differential diagnosis maps and to review the clinical findings for a variety of injuries and conditions. Readers should use the blank templates provided in Appendices A and B to create differential maps for these cases. This collection of cases is left open-ended by design. The goal is to provide learners with realistic scenarios in order to practice their differential diagnosis skills. The authors derived these cases from their own clinical practices; the names and ages for each case have been altered to protect patient privacy. Enjoy!

Paper Patient: Knee Pain in a Soccer Player

History

Robert is a 21-year-old recreational soccer player who reports to the athletic trainer with intermittent knee pain. He states that his knee is painful after exercising or if he is seated for prolonged periods of time. Robert describes pain with squatting motions, walking up and down stairs, and moving from flexion to extension (eg, getting up from sitting to standing).

Winterstein AP, Clark SV. *The Athletic Trainer's Guide to Differential Diagnosis (pp 389-396).*

Robert also states he has pain with walking for long periods of time. He denies any acute mechanism of injury. He states that the knee has not been swollen and he has no night pain.

Physical Exam

Robert's AROM is WNL and pain free. PROM is WNL with a normal end feel. All of the performed ligamentous exams (varus, valgus, anterior and posterior drawer, and Lachman's) are negative for laxity and pain. There is no joint effusion and no tenderness to the joint line. Robert is tender to palpation at the inferior pole of the patella and at the mid substance of the patellar tendon. There is no discernible crepitus. The patellar apprehension test is negative. His lower extremity neurovascular exam is normal. His foot alignment and arch height are WNL. No abnormalities in lower limb alignment are noted. Thomas test for hip flexor tightness is positive. Ober's test for iliotibial band tightness is also positive.

Paper Patient: Hip Pain in a Football Player

History

Adam is a 17-year-old male who comes off the football field complaining of right hip pain towards his groin. He was tackled by a player who landed on top of his back while his right hip was in external rotation, abduction and was pushed into extension. He walked off the field of his own accord and was limping a bit, but not more than expected for coming off the field after being injured. He denies previous injury to the hip. He denies numbness or tingling. His pain rating was 3 to 4/10 on the visual analog scale of 0 to 10.

Physical Exam

Adam was taken into the locker room for a quick exam, and he has ROM WNL. FABER test is painful. MMT in sitting is 4/5 for internal and external rotation. Supine hip flexion testing reveals 5/5 strength. The patient was given crutches and an appointment was made for the following morning for radiographs.

Paper Patient: Ankle Injury in a College Student

History

Melissa is a 29-year-old graduate student who reports spraining her ankle 8 days ago while stepping off the curb on her way to class. She describes an inversion mechanism of injury. She was seen at her local urgent care and was told she had normal radiographs. For the past week, she has been wearing a compression wrap. She indicates that she has been staying off the ankle and now has significant stiffness and pain. She had done no structured rehabilitation or self care. She notes that she still has swelling on the lateral aspect of the ankle and has pain with ambulation and ADLs.

Physical Exam

Melissa's AROM at the ankle reveals limitations in dorsiflexion. PROM is WNL with normal end feel but painful at the extremes of motion. She is tender to palpation over the anterior talofibular ligament and the calcaneofibular ligament. The anterior drawer test is positive for pain but equal bilaterally for laxity. The inversion stress test is positive for pain; Ant Drawer test is positive for pain but equal bilaterally for laxity. MMT reveals 4/5 strength in resisted eversion (painful) and 5/5 strength in all other planes of motion. There is visible ecchymosis and some pitting edema is noted along the lateral aspect of the ankle. Her neurovascular exam is normal.

Paper Patient: Lower Leg/Ankle Pain in a Runner

History

Pete is a very active 29-year-old runner who is in training for several competitive events. He reports that he has had pain (5/10) in his lower leg behind his ankle in the region of his Achilles for about a week and has noticed some discomfort for about 2 weeks. He had a painful run 3 days ago and noticed swelling in the tendon area when he was changing his socks. Pete runs about 6/7 days per week and has had to cut back in the past couple of weeks due to gradually increasing discomfort. He currently runs about

40 miles per week, down from his normal 60. He does report a tough hill workout recently, but states that it was not out of the ordinary for his training. He has been cross training for a few days due to his pain with running.

Physical Exam

Pete has visible swelling along the distal Achilles tendon. There is tenderness to palpation over the Achilles at the insertion with palpable crepitus. Pete's PROM is WNL with normal end feel, but soft tissue tightness at the gastrocnemius/soleus complex is noted at end range. Strength is evaluated by MMT and is 5/5 all planes of the ankle; pain is noted with resisted plantar flexion. His foot alignment is WNL. He has a normal foot and ankle exam (no ligamentous issues or joint swelling).

Paper Patient: Foot Pain in a Recreational Runner

History

Adam is a 21-year-old runner. He presented to clinic with vague pain in his left foot. He reports that the pain feels better in the morning and then returns as he progresses through the day. The pain runs towards his toes and the ball of the foot. He describes a burning and occasional numbness. He reports that he recently changed his footwear, and that the toe box may be a bit tight in his new shoes. He has had to stop his afternoon runs, but still tries to run in the morning before the pain gets worse. He has not changed his running mileage or surface recently. He does not wear orthotics.

Physical Exam

His physical exam reveals that Adam is tender over forefoot region, and he has specific soreness between the second and third metatarsals. Adam has a pes planus foot alignment with calcaneal eversion. There is pain with MMT for dorsiflexion of the ankle and with extension of the toes. The squeeze test of the forefoot is positive for vague pain. Long axis compression of the metatarsals is negative, as are bump and Tinel's tests. A long second toe is noted.

Paper Patient: Shoulder Pain Following Exercise Classes

History

Allison is a 40-year-old active female who comes with a 6-month history of right shoulder pain. She has been following a home exercise video for strength with a lot of overhead activity. She did this every day for 18 days, and as she was doing a push-up, she felt something in her shoulder. She has had to lift boxes for moving and has been in awkward positions with the shoulder. She gets numbness and tingling sometimes in the shoulder with certain positions. She has a deep, horrible ache, and she can't lie on that side. She experiences clicking in her shoulder on a regular basis. She denies previous injury to her shoulder. She has had issues at the elbow before. She thought that by now she would be better, but she is not.

Physical Exam

Allison's active motion at the shoulder is 170 degrees left and 153 degrees on the right for flexion. Abduction is 164 degrees left and 152 degrees with pain starting at 135 degrees on the right. Apley's for internal rotation is T3 on the left and T10 with pain on the right. External rotation at 90 degrees of abduction measures 98 degrees left and 104 degrees right. Internal rotation in the sleeper stretch position is 50 degrees on the left and 10 degrees with pain on the right. Her MMTs are as follows: external rotation in neutral 5/5 bilaterally and pain on the right. Internal rotation in neutral was 5/5 bilaterally with pain on the right. Supraspinatus i 5/5 bilaterally with no pain. Deltoid was 5/5 bilaterally with pain on the right.

The patient has intact sensation of upper extremity dermatomes and intact function of upper extremity myotomes. Positive Neer's, Hawkins Kennedy, and cross-over tests, negative Speed's, negative full can, positive empty can, and patient demonstrates capsular end feel with passive motion. The patient has both a positive crank and O'Brien's test.

Paper Patient: Wrist Pain in a Club Tennis Player

History

Alan is a 25-year-old graduate student who plays on a club tennis team. He reports to clinic for evaluation with left wrist pain that has been present (on and off) for 4 to 5 months. Alan is a right-hand dominant player who describes a sharp pain toward his distal ulna with movement. He cannot recall an acute MOI. He notices pain with ADLs as well as with tennis activities. Alan reports that lifting, grasping, and bearing weight on his palm are causing pain in the wrist.

Physical Exam

Alan's AROM of the wrist is WNL but he does report pain (3/10) with wrist extension. His PROM is WNL with normal end feel, but he again reports pain (4/10) with wrist extension. A clicking sound/sensation is noted with extension and flexion of the wrist. He is tender to palpation over the ulnar collateral ligament (UCL) and the triangular fibrocartilage complex (TFCC). MMT reveals 4/5 and painful in wrist extension and 4/5 and painful in wrist flexion. There is no bony tenderness, and Alan's neurovascular exam is normal.

Paper Patient: Right Side/Rib Pain in an Ultimate Player

History

Tom was injured 1 week ago while playing Ultimate. He reports on acute MOI when he jumped up to catch a disc and the right side of his rib cage was struck by another player's shoulder. He had immediate chest wall pain. He stopped playing and rested for a couple of days. At that point, he felt better, so he played in another game and noticed pain (5/10) while playing. This pain worsened after stopping. He reports difficulty finding a comfortable sleeping position, pain with deep breaths, and he is unable to exercise. Tom explains that he has varying levels of pain (4 to 7/10) when he moves his trunk, laughs, coughs, or takes deep breaths.

Physical Exam

Tom reports pain (5/10) along the right side of his rib cage during shoulder ROM. AROM of the upper extremity is WNL but painful with full overhead motions. Active lateral bending of the trunk reveals pain (5/10) in the right side (both directions). He is tender to palpation at the area near the seventh rib area of costochondral junction. There is a small area of ecchymosis over the tender location. Full inspiration and expiration produces 3/10 pain. There are no palpable defects and he has a normal respiration rate (16 breaths per minute).

Paper Patient: Elbow Pain in a Youth Baseball Pitcher

History

Ian is a 13-year-old Little League pitcher who complains of left elbow pain. He is left-hand dominant. He just switched teams this summer from a recreational league to a more competitive league. He is pitching twice as much as he is accustomed to, and the pain started shortly after the start of the third week. When he was younger, he did gymnastics and his mom reports that he was always doing handstands. He denies previous injury to the left elbow. He notes that sometimes his elbow doesn't feel quite right when he goes from flexion to extension of the elbow. It is kind of like a catch with pain. He notices that his elbow looks swollen sometimes after practice. He doesn't have numbness, but when the pain is bad, he states that it kind of tingles.

Physical Exam

On physical exam, the patient is tender to palpation at the medial epicondyle and flexor mass. There is no flexor mass tightness compared to the right side with palpation. There is a trace to one effusion at the medial elbow. Tap testing is negative for the ulnar nerve, as was nerve tension testing. He has pain with MMT for flexion of the wrist with the elbow flexed, as well as with pronation and less with supination. Forearm and biceps and triceps strength was WNL. He did experience a catch-like sensation as well as pain with triceps testing. The patient has pain with valgus stress at the elbow and some tingling.

Paper Patient: Blow to the Face in a Field Hockey Game

History

Amanda is a 21-year-old field hockey player who was hit in the face by an opponent's hockey stick. Your questioning reveals that the blow was to the cheek area on the left side. She reports that she has severe pain 8/10 on the visual analog scale of 0 to 10. Her jaw feels like it isn't closing correctly. Her nose is bleeding profusely and she complains of double vision and numbness in the lip and cheek region.

Physical Exam

Your physical exam on the field reveals no tenderness over the cervical spine. She has tenderness to palpation over the upper jaw on the left. The eyes are WNL. The patient is bleeding from the left nostril and it won't stop. You deem it necessary to transport the athlete right away.

Paper Patient: Back Pain in a Football Player

History

Mike is a 16-year-old football player who complains of neck pain and numbness and tingling that runs down to the fingers on the right side. He tackled an opponent and his neck bent to the side as he wrapped the running back with his arms to tackle him.

Physical Exam

Your exam reveals no tenderness to palpation over the spinous processes of the cervical spine. The patient has pain with active motion cervical flexion to the left. He also notes numbness and tingling with this. MMT reveals weakness in the myotomes of the upper extremity. There is loss of sensation in the dermatomes as well. You have the athlete sit while you document your findings. You repeat the testing of the upper quarter screen and note improvement.

A

Differential Diagnosis Templates

Winterstein AP, Clark SV. *The Athletic Trainer's Guide to Differential Diagnosis (pp 397-399).*

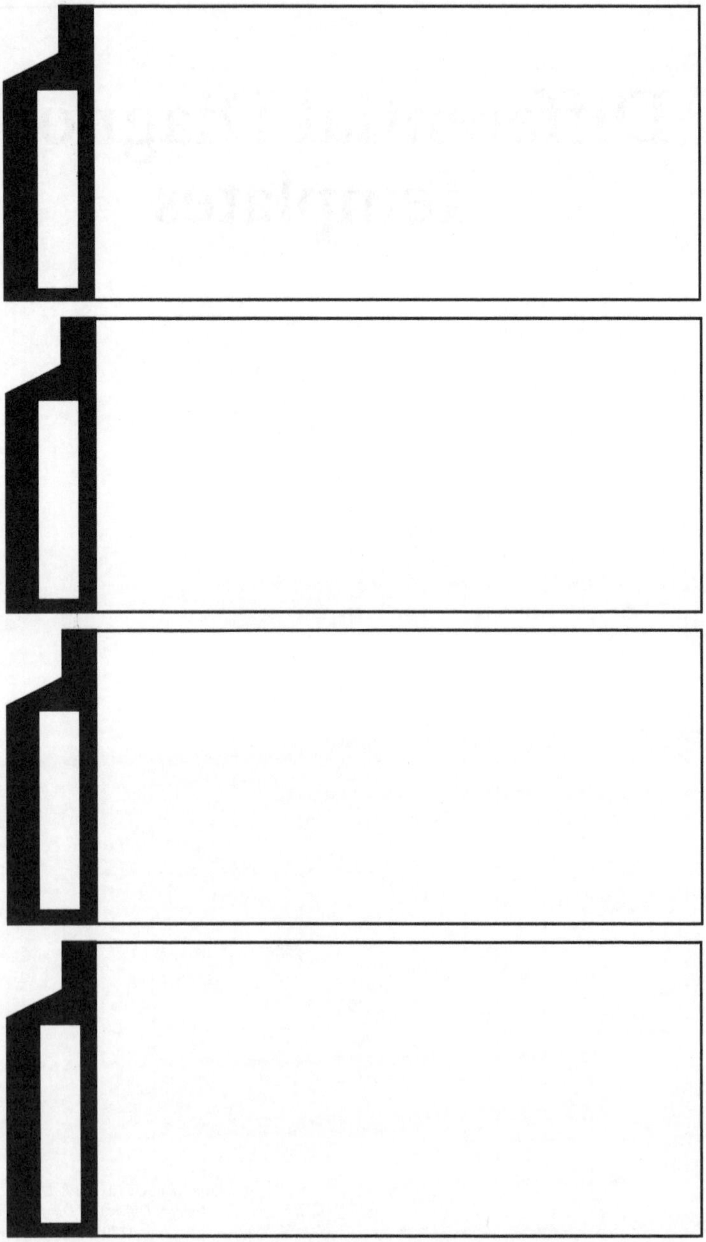

B

Clinical Findings Templates

Winterstein AP, Clark SV. *The Athletic Trainer's Guide to Differential Diagnosis (pp 401-403).*

HISTORY	MECHANISM OF INJURY	EVALUATION ESSENTIALS

KEY FINDINGS	DIAGNOSTIC EVIDENCE

HISTORY	MECHANISM OF INJURY	EVALUATION ESSENTIALS

KEY FINDINGS	DIAGNOSTIC EVIDENCE

C

Bibliography

Each chapter in the *Athletic Trainer's Guide to Differential Diagnosis: A Visual Learning Approach* was written with appropriate referencing of current literature. Special attention was given to citing appropriate sources for the Diagnostic Evidence section (when available) in the Clinical Findings of each injury. However, much of the clinical findings information originated from the authors combined 48 years of clinical experience as athletic trainers. Over the course of a long career of teaching and clinical practice we recognize that we have been influenced by many quality athletic training and sports medicine textbooks. While these textbooks may not have been directly cited we wish to thoughtfully acknowledge their influence on the body of knowledge in the athletic training domain.

Anderson MK, Hall SJ, Martin M. *Foundations of Athletic Training: Prevention, Assessment, and Management.* Philadelphia, PA: Lippincott Williams & Wilkins; 2008.

Cook C, Hegedus EJ. *Orthopedic Physical Examination Tests: An Evidence-Based Approach.* Upper Saddle River, NJ: Prentice-Hall; 2008.

Higgins M. *Therapeutic Exercise: From Theory to Practice.* Philadelphia, PA: FA Davis Company; 2011.

Houglum PA. *Therapeutic Exercise for Musculoskeletal Injuries.* 3rd ed. Champaign, IL: Human Kinetics; 2010.

Magee DJ. *Orthopaedic Physical Assessment.* Elsevier Health Sciences; 2008.

Prentice WE. *Principles of Athletic Training: A Competency-Based Approach.* 14th ed. New York, NY: McGraw Hill; 2011.

Winterstein AP, Clark SV. *The Athletic Trainer's Guide to Differential Diagnosis (pp 405–406).*

Shultz SJ, Houglum PA, Perrin DH. *Examination of Musculoskeletal Injuries.* 2nd ed. Champaign, IL: Human Kinetics; 2005.

Starkey C, ed. *Athletic Training and Sports Medicine: An Integrated Approach.* 5th ed. Jones & Bartlett Publishers; 2012.

Starkey C, Brown SD, Ryan JL. *Examination of Orthopedic and Athletic Injuries.* Philadelphia, PA: FA Davis Company; 2010.

Index